ENDORSEMENTS

I want to thank Sophia for this insightful sharing of her life and experiences along this glorious Siddha Path. This book provides an excellent resource of inspiration on many levels. Sharing is a sacred practice an excellent opportunity on the part of a devotee to give back for the light that has been brought into our lives by the Guru's grace in our lives. This book is a wonderful example of seva on the part of Sophia, because it is so important to encourage others to seize this golden opportunity in their lives and follow a path such as Siddha Yoga. Each of these sharings help us to bring this power into our lives and urge us on and enrich all aspects of our lives and return to our true divine nature.

-Ken Anirudha Van Skaik, Siddha Yoga Devotee, B.A. History

Life's journey is such an amazing adventure! Sophia captures the essence of that journey through her personal story of trials and growth forging a path for others and revealing the importance of awaking through our own personal expression of inspiration. Wonderful read!

-Carrie-Anne D'Angelo, Token Rock Co-founder and author of Notes From Within

Sophia Paul is an inspiration and blessing to those wanting to learn about living a peaceful yogic lifestyle. She provides thoughtful insight along with practical knowledge that will resonate with people of all levels of experience. This book will inspire the reader to bring out the beauty in their lives through yoga.

-Christina McDevitt, CC Licensed and certified Heal Your Life® Instructor Certified Life Purpose and Career Coach

An inspirational book which, with skill and sensitivity, leads the reader to help transform daily life into an extraordinary adventure. Sophia has been a mentor and teacher to me for many years and has changed my life forever. There is never enough of this kind of inspired material!

-Jennifer Kachnic, CCMT, Certified Reiki Practitioner,
CANINE WELLNESS, LLC, Author of Your Dog's
Golden Years - A Manual for Senior Dog Care
- Including Alternative and Complementary Options

It's Not About Putting Your Foot Behind Your Ear

An Inspiring Journey of Transformation Through YOGA

Sophia S Paul

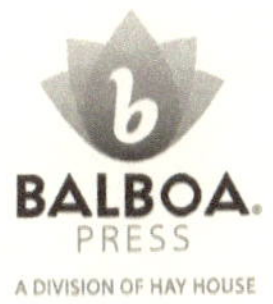

Balboa Press books may be ordered through booksellers or by contacting:

Balboa Press
A Division of Hay House
1663 Liberty Drive
Bloomington, IN 47403
www.balboapress.com
1-(877) 407-4847

Editors: Mira S K Paul and Lauren Wise
Photographer: Sophia Paul, Bastian Paul, Stephanie Perlowski

Includes bibliography and recommended reading list.
www.sophiapaul.com
www.royalyogabailey.com
www.omshantiyogawear.com

ISBN: 978-1-4525-3995-9 (e)
ISBN: 978-1-4525-3996-6 (sc)
ISBN: 978-1-4525-3997-3 (hc)

Library of Congress Control Number: 2011917813

Printed in the United States of America

Balboa Press rev. date: 10/26/2011

DEDICATION

This book is dedicated especially to my children Manuel, Kevin, and Mira, and grandchildren Bastian and Lena. All of you are and have been the greatest inspiration to me. From the moment you were born (maybe even before that) you all helped me become who I am. The strength of our family lies in believing in each other, sticking together when times get tough, and always being there for each other. I love you with all my heart.

A big thank you to everyone who has ever touched my life. All of you contributed to my journey. It is my deepest wish that I have touched yours as well and that sharing my story will be an inspiration to you when you most need it; when you feel that you have come to a point in your life where things appear hopeless. Maybe my musings will help you through to see the silver lining! May you all be blessed.

Thank you to NATURE for always helping me see the bigger picture and to believe in Greatness and Wonder. It is my promise to continue taking care of you the best way I can, to nurture and protect you with all my strength.

Namaste—The Divine in Me honors the Divine in You

ACKNOWLEDGEMENTS

A special THANK YOU to

Mira for your support, input and knowledge and giving me the confidence to move forward with my book;

Jenny for walking the "Author's Path" together with me and for sharing all our resources;

Christina for lifting me up and making me laugh when things seem dull and for our "water cooler talk" (you know what I mean);

Colleen Deffner for being my long-term yogini and supporter for all my "causes";

Lauren for your great work and patience.

FOREWORD

As a physician, as well as a published author, it was a double honor for me to write the foreword to this book. When I first started my medical practice over 45 years ago, little was known about alternative medicine. That's not to say that little was known about yoga; it's been around for well over 5,000 years, though in America it was little practices and certainly not considered a medical alternative.

But "medical alternative" is perhaps a bad term. Although yoga has proven to have powerful healing qualities, no yoga teacher or practitioner would suggest that yoga replace good medical advice. On the other hand, no knowledgeable physician would doubt that yoga would be a good adjunct to his or her therapy program.

There is no doubt in the minds of modern physicians that yoga is a healing system in both theory and practice—it's a combination of controlled breathing exercises, physical postures, and meditation.

A survey released in May 2004 by the National Center for Complementary and Alternative Medicine indicated that yoga was the fifth most commonly used Complimentary Alternative

Medicine therapy in the United States, by adults aged 18 and older who used this type of medicine.

So how does yoga work to combat disease? Yoga is a mind-body intervention that reduces the health effects of generalized stress, a serious component of most physical and psychological problems and diseases. Furthermore, yoga calms the nervous system and balances the body, mind, and spirit. Its practitioners and most knowledgeable physicians believe that yoga is able to prevent many specific diseases and maladies.

For example, yoga has been used to lower blood pressure, reduce stress, and improve coordination, flexibility, concentration, sleep, and digestion. All these factors have powerful influences on both health and disease recovery. People use yoga for a great variety of health conditions, and to achieve physical and mental fitness and relaxation. There is growing evidence to suggest that yoga enhances stress-coping mechanisms and mind-body awareness.

I mentioned earlier that being asked to write this foreword was a double honor for me, being a physician and author of more than 40 published books. Most of my books are self-help health oriented so this book especially caught my interest, not just for its excellent health information, but because it reads like a novel. It is in fact a memoir of the author's own travel through a life filled with adventure, love and love lost, disappointments, and serious pitfalls, and most importantly, pulling herself up from devastating low points in her life as a single mother without an income. Yoga played a huge role in her rebounding to new successes and a fulfilled life.

She proves that yoga is not just for the young, and as she states it is not just about "putting your foot behind your ear." Yoga is a powerful source of inspiration, a tool for building self-esteem, a force that can assist you in achieving your loftiest goals. In her 30 plus years as a yoga practitioner and teacher, she has learned to appreciate the power of the yogic lifestyle and has made it her obligation to pass on this vast knowledge.

Yoga was originally developed as a method of discipline to help people reach spiritual enlightenment. However, yoga also strongly influences psychological and physical health while enhancing focus, which leads to professional success and character that leads on to social successes.

With all its positive factors, it's no wonder that more than 13 million adults used yoga between 2002 and 2007, and that number has increased by approximately three million people since then. In addition, that same survey also found that more than 1.5 million children used yoga.

Just a few of the health conditions people find help for through yoga including anxiety disorders and stress, asthma, high blood pressure, and depression, as well as part of a general health regimen designed to achieve physical, and mental fitness and health.

There are very few contraindications to the judicial practice of yoga—it is generally considered safe for healthy people when practiced appropriately with trained supervision and has few side effects. However, people with certain medical conditions should avoid some yoga practices. For example, people with disc disease of the spine, extremely high or low blood pressure, glaucoma, retinal detachment, fragile or atherosclerotic arteries, a risk of blood clots, ear problems, severe osteoporosis, joints of limited motion, or cervical spondylitis should avoid some of the more extreme poses.

If you are considering yoga for the first time, let me suggest certain precautions:

Do not use yoga as a replacement for conventional care or to postpone seeing a doctor about a medical problem; yoga is a great adjunct to conventional medicine, and may indeed replace certain conventional medical treatments, but these changes should be made *with* your medical advisor's knowledge.

If you have a medical condition, or under treatment for any physical problems, always consult with your health care provider before starting yoga.

Don't hesitate to ask about the physical demands of the type of yoga in which you are interested, as well as the training and experience of the yoga teacher you are considering.

Consult with your health care providers about any new, or complementary and alternative practices you are considering. By the same token let your yoga instructor know about any medical problems you may have, providing a full picture of what you do to manage your health. This will ensure coordinated and safe care between your physician and yoga instructor.

Meditation in medicine

Siddhartha Gautama, better known as the Buddha, declared 2500 years ago that suffering is subjective and can be reduced through self-awareness. Today, a growing number of American doctors and healthcare workers are utilizing Buddha's principles in treatment of their patients. In hospitals and clinics meditation is increasingly being presented as a method of stress reduction and to help patients better cope with the physical pain and mental strain associated with many medical conditions, including heart disease, stroke, post traumatic stress, and even HIV infection. Research shows meditation's soothing effects can be detected in arterial walls and in brain imaging.

Meditation is the act of dis-identifying from inner thought flow and concentrating on calming and healing. Doctors help patients detach from their pain and anxieties to cultivate a connection between the mind and the body through meditation. The aim is to assist people in taking better care of themselves through a daily discipline of meditation and relaxation. Doctors refer patients to meditation programs and practitioners for any number of diseases and disorders, including heart disease, anxiety and panic, job or family stress, chronic pain, cancer, headaches, sleep disturbances, type A behavior, high blood pressure, fatigue, skin disorders, and numerous other maladies. Meditation has helped recent military veterans deal with post-traumatic stress disorder. Meditation has more recently been used to treat eating disorders, alcoholism, psoriasis, and even impotence.

Relaxation and reducing stress through meditation may also reduce artery blockage and the risk of heart attack and stroke, according to a study released by the American Heart Association's journal. Another recent pilot study, published in the NeuroReport, by Sara Lazar, Ph.D., a Harvard research fellow in psychology at

Massachusetts General Hospital, in Boston, suggests meditation activates specific regions of the brain that may influence heart and breathing rates. The usual, fight-or-flight brain response liberates adrenaline and is stressful to the body, but during meditation the brain acts to quiet the body through concentrated breathing or word repetition, evoking a relaxation response that minimizes the harmful effects of stress. A growing body of research shows that meditation has a discernible effect on the brain that promotes various types of health and well-being.

More than six million Americans are now being referred for meditation, and other mind-body therapies by conventional health care providers, according to a report released by Harvard Medical School. Some more progressive insurance companies, such as Blue Cross/Blue Shield in Massachusetts and other more enlightened states like Oregon and California, are actually now paying for all or part of these programs.

Othniel Seiden, M.D.

CONTENTS

PART 2

PART 3

PART 4

PART 5

PART 6

Chapter 24

One fresh thought, one change of heart, one leap of faith, can change your life forever.

~ Robert Holden

STILLNESS

When I completely quiet my mind, the pace of my world slows down and a space opens, appearing as if a heavy fog slowly lifts, Divine light enters and I can connect with the sacredness of my soul—finding answers to my most profound questions in the stillness of my heart. SSP

INTRODUCTION

So you really thought that yoga was about putting your foot behind your ear?

It's not! This book is about dispelling the myths about yoga being only for the young, fit and flexible as well as that one has to become a Buddhist/Hindu or that one will be converted into a different belief system in order to benefit from yoga. I want to encourage and inspire you to step out of your comfort zone and try something new—that weird thing called yoga that is so much more than just the poses we all have seen before. It takes courage, a sense of purpose, awareness and a willingness to allow yourself to go with the flow and to be open to the beauty of the present moment. Yoga is a lifestyle, a journey and it is suitable for everyone at any age.

Attitude is everything is one of my life mottos; this book is a testimonial about positive thinking and making the best out of every situation, resulting in living a rich, vibrant, inspired life.

It is my sincere wish and hope to inspire and empower people of all ages, shapes, and backgrounds to enhance their existence through living mindfully and with an open heart by integrating the ancient principles of yoga into their daily lives. It is meant to put those at ease who are looking for alternatives to bringing their lives into balance but thought that yoga was not for them. And last but not least I wish to inspire you to always look towards the new door opening rather than the one that just closed right in front of you by staying mindful in the present moment.

This book is NOT a textbook about yoga poses or a meditation guide per se; there are plenty of those on the market.

This is my personal inspiring story how my journey and yogic path started and extended over several countries and continents. It is about the development and transformation through the practice of yoga with all its components, physically, mentally, emotionally and spiritually; a story from the early beginnings and discoveries of the life-saving benefits of yoga during some major challenges in my life including a devastating divorce, being stranded in a foreign country, dealing with severe illnesses in my family to my personal journey of becoming a certified yoga instructor.

I am sharing yoga success stories from some of my students who never believed that yoga was for them, only to discover that in some instances it turned their lives around 100%. Included also are stories from people who do live inspired and passionate lives, why they are doing what they are doing and how they got there. Bolded yoga terms throughout the book are simply defined in a back index.

My 30 plus years of experience as a yoga practitioner/instructor have given me a deep understanding and appreciation of a yogic lifestyle and how the focus on living an inspired life opens up new spectacular venues of a life lived in vibrant health and well-being.

I feel it is my obligation to share these experiences with as many people as I can.

Namaste

NOTE TO THE READER

I am glad your path has led you to this book. The simple fact that your journey directed you here and our paths crossed is a sign that your soul is telling you to take a look at other possibilities, to open yourself up to living an inspired life full of mindfulness and presence. Please feel free to read this book with a notebook at your side; copy down anything that may inspire you or jot down your own thoughts into your journal. Start your own inspirational writing: do it daily, get in the habit and be ready to experience a blissful journey towards your very own inspired life!

I am sending you blessings of abundance and happiness through each and every word and page of my book. All you have to do is allow them to flow into your life, shower you and envelop you day by day, minute by minute, second by second.

PART 1

"The soul that moves in the world of the senses and yet keeps the senses in harmony... finds rest in quietness."

~ ***Bhagavad Gita***

Only Breath

Not Christian or Jew or Muslim, not Hindu
Buddhist, Sufi, or Zen. Not any religion

or cultural system. I am not from the East
or the West, not out of the ocean or up

from the ground, not natural or ethereal, not
composed of elements at all. I do not exist,

am not an entity in this world or in the next,
did not descend from Adam and Eve or any

origin story. My place is placeless, a trace
of the traceless. Neither body or soul.

I belong to the beloved, have seen the two
worlds as one and that one call to and know,

first, last, outer, inner, only that
breath breathing human being.

From *Essential Rumi*
by Coleman Barks

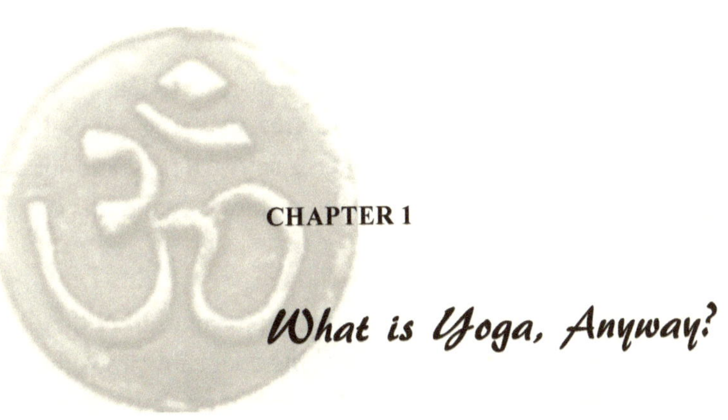

CHAPTER 1

What is Yoga, Anyway?

Yoga is not just about being able to put your foot behind your ear, although the physical aspect of flexibility is important—just recently I fell off the kitchen counter onto the tile floor, and my flexibility, strength and quick reaction probably saved me from a broken hip. But there is so much more to yoga than just the poses that we all know and see.

The most important part of yoga is to learn the ability to stay centered and focused—no matter what—to allow our minds to remain calm and at peace in the midst of tumult, chaos and challenges. Being connected to our body and mind through the breath is one of the greatest gifts we can give to ourselves.

Yoga is a lifestyle; not just an exercise. Yoga is to be practiced on and off the mat during our daily lives. Through yoga we can learn to act as the observer, to stay detached from the situation, or challenge such as our negative thoughts or energy, therefore achieving emotional healing, an opening of the heart and calming of the mind.

"Making peace with our bodies through the practice of yoga" is one of the key concepts that Christina Sell conveys to us in her inspiring book *Yoga from the Inside Out* (pg 61). She further states that, "...**asana practice** could transform our relationship with our bodies, helping us to create peace and assisting our soul in its evolution…to breathe when things get intense, to soften where we are hard and to strengthen where we are weak" (pg 83). Sell reminds us that **hatha yoga**, at its roots, is a spiritual practice, not to be confused with a competition, fashion show or a popularity contest (pg 105). Well said, Christina!

Many of my students confirm that after their yoga class they realize they had not spent a moment thinking about any problems or issues that seemed so important when they first walked into the room. How is this possible? It's actually simple; we give our minds something else to do, such as focusing on breathing and the correct facilitation of the according yoga movements. As much as our minds like to stay busy and jump from subject to subject, when we take control and give it something to do we can rest assured the mind will obey.

There is an ancient saying that "the mind is like a raging elephant," and slowly through some helpful tools (such as meditation, **mantras, mudras**) we can learn how to put reins on what is also called the restless monkey mind.

We will experience a deep sense of peace and relaxation by fusing together three things: staying mentally focused, paying attention to the correct alignment, and being fully present in our body while practicing yoga postures that are initiated by breath. We then can apply those same qualities to everything we do and encounter in our lives. Being fully aware in the present moment is the key. Most of us are so used to constant multi-tasking; we watch TV while we eat dinner, while talking on the phone and reading a book.

As Thich Nhat Hanh says, "When we are mindful, deeply in touch with the present moment, our understanding of what is going on deepens, and we begin to be filled with acceptance, joy, peace and love." Another saying is, "When you wash the dishes, wash the dishes; when you drink tea, drink tea; when you watch the sun rise, watch the sun rise." What does that mean? At the tender age of 11 my daughter once said to me, "Mom, to you everything is a meditation." It was the best compliment someone could have ever given to me. This is the way I try to live my life: Living in the present moment. It is all that we will ever have. The past is gone and the future has not yet arrived, but this very moment is there for us to make it into anything we want. We have the option to laugh, to appreciate, allow, enjoy or—to ignore it, worry about what may be, being angry over what has been. We cannot change the past nor the future, so why not fully embrace the here and now?

Richard Faulds (Kripalu Yoga) states, "...the essence of meditation is a state of deep inner absorption that can occur in either the flow of yoga postures or in moments of physical stillness." And Yogi Amrit Desai once said, "Yesterday is dead. Tomorrow isn't been born. We can only live in the present."

When I was being taught **Vipassana meditation**, I was guided to experience the stillness that naturally arises in the moments between the in and out breaths. Eckhart Tolle recommends becoming aware of the spaces between words. He says that stillness brings awareness of silence, and it's in the silence that we can experience being fully awake. Consciousness is beyond thought activity. There's more power in the gaps between the words than in the words themselves.

"In the sweet territory of silence we touch the mystery. It's the place of reflection and contemplation, and it's the place where we can connect with the deep knowing, to the deep wisdom way." —Angeles Arrien

When I look back at my life I can clearly see how yoga—just like the spine in my body—is the central channel (or ***shushumna*** in yogic terms). It is the constant, the straight line that always keeps me focused and aligned with what matters in life. As I keep my spine straight I keep my alignment, if I slump, all I have to do is notice and make a small correction. It is the same with all that happens during our lifetime. Awareness is key. The shushumna, or central channel, is also related to our breath, so by keeping the spine straight, the breath (or ***prana***, life force) can flow freely. Remember when we were little and mom said when we were upset to "just take a deep breath?" Well she was right; taking deep slow breaths has an immediate effect on our nervous system. Our main **chakras** (energy centers) are aligned along the spine as well, and if they spin freely and openly we have a better chance of a healthy life, physically, mentally, and emotionally. Of course, keeping everything nicely aligned would be something in a perfect world. For most of us there are dips, valleys, highs, wavering. Life would be boring if it was otherwise, but sometimes we feel overwhelmed, losing focus, feeling alone, abandoned, hurt. Keeping that straight line in our minds, allowing it to reel us back into alignment and to focus is the ultimate goal.

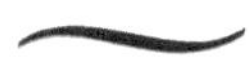

The spiritual journey is not about becoming perfect but to live every moment with awareness, mindfulness and integrity. SSP

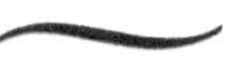

One of the physical goals of yoga of course is alignment in every pose. Through proper alignment we achieve flexibility without hurting ourselves. The same applies to the mental/emotional goals: If we align with a higher source—whatever that may be for each one of us, for some it may be Jesus, for others—Allah,

Muhammad, Great Spirit, Buddha, Krishna—we will always have something to turn to *or* return to. Aligning, allowing, focus.

Once again, perceiving yoga as a safe space in its entirety, where we accept ourselves and others with all our differences, worldviews, capabilities, bodies and beliefs, creates a sanctuary that we might not find elsewhere. "What if we truly knew, in every cell of our bodies, that we are lovable exactly as we are in the moment?" Christina Sell (*Yoga From The Inside Out,* pg 128) suggests.

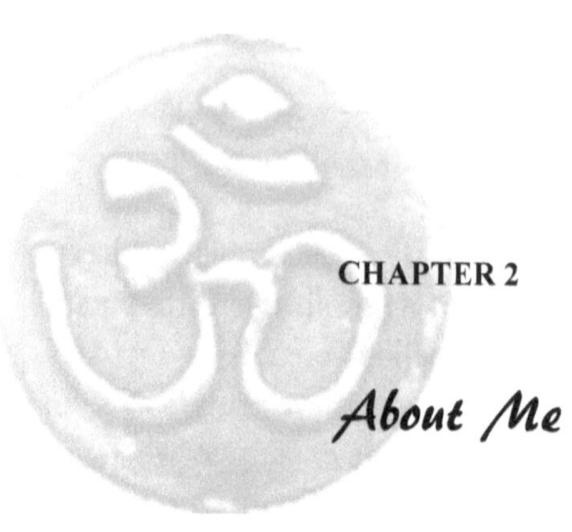

CHAPTER 2

About Me

On a beautiful sunny Saturday afternoon at 2 pm, I was born in an idyllic small village at the base of an ancient hill adorned with medieval castle ruins. Of course, in those days the entire family was present for this magical moment. The mid-wife was taking care of me while I was kicking and screaming (yes, that is me, right) and for some reason my foot got caught in the bow of her apron while she turned around, and it ripped me off the table. My beloved Pate (that is a German name for godfather) caught me and saved my tiny little precious life. Ever since, we have had a very close relationship with each other.

I grew up with mom and dad, aunt and uncle, cousin and grandparents all under one big roof in a beautiful garden full of vegetables, fruit, flowers, fruit trees, chickens, pigs, goats, geese. What a paradise it was. I had the biggest sandbox one could ever imagine, there was a "garden" house where Grandma told me stories and we played. I cooked a "flower" meal for her and baked sand cakes, and she "ate" it all. When the weather was not so nice I spent most of my time with grandma, cooking, baking and watching her sew clothes for me.

The entire family went on Sunday walks, me riding on Pate's shoulders, smearing blueberries all over his head, but he loved me anyways—unconditional love!!!

Adventures

However, there was a particular day when I thought that beautiful little world of mine was too small, and I decided to explore. I think I was three- or four-years-old. So I packed my dad's rucksack that was so large it dragged on the ground behind me, took his guitar (don't ask me why), put my boots on and my "Tiroler Hut" (a hat typical for the Tyrol area in Northern Italy) and left. Nobody noticed. I got about a quarter of a mile just past the neighbor's house when the neighbors saw me and casually asked where I was going. "Exploring the world," was my equally casual answer. Well, they asked me if I would want some cookies and milk before embarking on this long journey, and, sure enough, that sounded like a great idea and I went inside, forgot about the journey and enjoyed being spoiled. My parents showed up shortly thereafter, surprised of course but not even mad, just took me back home. So that is where my first big adventure ended, and my dream of the big wide world started.

My dad signed up with military, which meant that we had to move far, far away into an apartment complex. Life changed dramatically. No gardens, no sandbox to myself, no family except my mom and dad, and dad was gone most of the day on military assignments.

I couldn't wait for the six weeks of summer break when I was sent off to visit my grandparents, aunt and uncle again. Back in heaven, it seemed. How miserable I was when I had to go back "home;" in fact, it was NOT home at all. Home was where I was happy, and that was in my long-gone childhood paradise.

I was eight years old when my mom became pregnant with my brother. Things changed dramatically again. I was told that I really wasn't wanted in the first place, that all she wanted was a little boy with dark hair and not a bald, screaming little girl like me that looked like a "wet rat" (her words about me when I was born). Damage done… so I was the ugly undesirable one, barely tolerated.

It got worse when my brother was born, he, the "crowned prince" and I, Cinderella. I was basically nonexistent.

Days passed slowly but when it came time to go back to Grandma's home for the summer it was like a miracle. I was loved, taken care of, recognized. Life was good.

First Love and the Loss of It

When I was nine-years-old my neighborhood childhood friend spent his summer with his Grandma too, and we reconnected. We took walks up the ancient hill and sat on the ruins of the castle overlooking our little village, the wheat fields and meadows swaying below, holding hands and experiencing our first little love story. The summer ended and we both had to go back to the places that we hated. But oh well, life goes on, little kids grow up, go to school and do what most kids do: skip school, fail quizzes, get older, experiment with alcohol—for me, pretty bad, almost daily after school but only for a short period of time. Then I got involved with the local kayaking club. I had a purpose and a challenge again, a family structure. The caretaker's daughter and I became best friends. Her brother was cute too and we fell in love—madly. My days were filled with summer fests and bon fires and dancing at the river banks to "El Condor Pasa" by Simon and Garfunkel until well after midnight, and then we camped out under the stars.

Then again it happened, my parents moved us away. Again, I had to leave all my new friends. I had a nervous breakdown and ran away from the new school. They put me in therapy and I was allowed to go back to Unna to visit. I was happy, all of my old friends showed up at the train station and my love was there as well with a bouquet of roses for me. Needless to say, I felt good, accepted and wanted. What a great time I had kayaking again, partying, laughing, and belonging, but of course this all came to an end when I had to go back "home."

Very early in the morning is the best time to meditate; there is a special quality to the earliest morning hours, such as freshness, calmness, stillness.

All experienced meditators and yogis meditate at dawn, allowing space and presence in and being open to invite the power of the spirit of the rising sun to illuminate the heart of their soul. This special time of day when all is quiet will set the tone for the rest of your day. Conscious awareness and an open expectancy of the beauty and splendor of this day will make all the difference in the world of how miraculous your life journey unfolds.

The more detached I become and open to the outcome, the more I trust. The more I trust, the more I can let go and love. The more I love, the more I manifest. All of that eliminates fear, resulting in peace.
SSP

New Beginnings and Painful Endings

I convinced my parents that the school they put me in wasn't working out for me, and I wanted a job. So I started my education as a window dresser (this doesn't even exist anymore today) and made some more friends. But I missed my old clique terribly.

Again, I was allowed to go back for a weekend, but things had changed. My boyfriend did not show up at the train station this time—red flag. His sister, my best girlfriend, made excuses to protect me but I just knew. That same night there was a big party we went to and I saw him with another girl. I lost it—the old fear of rejection, not being wanted, and not being lovable came back full force. For some odd reason I had an empty syringe with me (my father was a diabetic and I took one of his needles) I don't even know why I had it with me; perhaps my subconscious already knew that there would be a big disappointment waiting for me that I knew I could not handle. I had heard that by squirting air into your vein you could commit suicide. I was drunk already, went to the bathroom and tried to hit the vein. Thank goodness I was too drunk to even hit it, and by the time I finally got it in my friend had found me, kicked in the bathroom door and ripped the syringe out of my arm before bringing me home with some friends. What a wakeup call! Was he worth it? What was I doing?

Back in Bonn with my parents I still was not happy in the new environment, until I met another guy and we dated. I got my new sense of belonging, being wanted and loved again. He had to serve in Hamburg and there was no question in my mind that I would go with him as the only one who loved me and cared about me. So off we went to Hamburg. I was mostly alone—again—as he had to stay on the military grounds of course. We broke up.

Family Life—Finally!

The next guy I met at work I thought was finally the right one. I got pregnant, and we got married. I was happy, and I was so looking forward to having my own family to nurture and love and care for, and do everything differently than the way I grew up.

Like all my pregnancies to come, this first one was wonderful. I enjoyed feeling this little life growing inside of me, dreaming about my future as a mom and wife, how wonderful our life would be together.

My little boy was born premature. We thought we would lose him as he was so tiny and he could not breathe on his own; his skin was bluish gray and they took him away right after he was born. No chance of bonding, no breastfeeding. They said his only chance of surviving would be if he were put into an incubator right away. He was only six weeks early, but in those days (some thirty-seven years ago) it WAS a big deal. Back then there was no knowledge of how important skin contact and breastfeeding is, especially for premies.

When everything we do is steeped in mindfulness and we learn how to communicate with the Divine through acceptance and gratitude, when coming deep from our hearts with full awareness and intensified by the power of desire, when we are ready to surrender to the moment then we are prepared for the power and simplicity of prayer. But we also have to be open and ready to receive. Prayer is simple and kind, never demanding or forceful. And sometimes it may take a long time, or our prayers go unanswered and we need to and we will understand in time that there is a reason for that also. SSP

So here I was alone, my little boy far away from me. They would not even let me touch him and I had to shuffle across the entire hospital to see him behind thick glass walls in his incubator.

I was still weak from two days of labor and the big incision, but I stood there for two hours before passing out. I found myself back in my room and hospital bed. The nurses were mad at me. I didn't care. As soon as I felt a little better, off I went again to see my child. Again, I stood behind the glass walls connecting with him in my thoughts. I did not think of it back then as a meditation, but now I know that's what it was. I forgot about pain, cold, loneliness, being dizzy from standing in the hallway for that long; all I could feel and think of was my love for my little son. On a spiritual level I told him that all would be ok, in my mind I caressed his little body, touched his little hands and kissed his tiny cheeks and sometimes, like a little miracle when I felt so close to him that I was certain it was not my imagination but real, that I was holding him, smelling the baby scent—then he moved just a tiny bit or lifted one tiny little finger.

Finally the nurses felt sorry for me, but I think they also admired me for my persistence and they set up a chair for me—still behind the glass walls but at least I could sit and stay a lot longer. Sometimes they even brought me my food there instead of into my room.

After a week it was time for me to leave the hospital. I dreaded that day and pleaded to be able to stay longer, but of course insurance would not pay for it anymore. In tears I left, feeling like I was abandoning my child. I communicated with him heart to heart. I sat down and in my mind I was with him, holding him, comforting him, and loving him. Was that meditation? I believe it was. It was being totally present, totally focused on this one little precious child of mine. I was neither hungry nor sleepy, I was in a deep state of meditation—I realize that now. I was not religious but I prayed almost constantly to make him grow stronger and stronger, and finally we succeeded. After six nerve-wracking weeks we could finally take him home. We made it!!

It was not quite all glory though. He still was very weak, and he would not eat. I had to squeeze the formula into his little mouth, and most of the time he fell asleep after a few moments. I was afraid; so afraid I might lose him after all. He did not gain weight as he was supposed to. At the next visit to the hospital they told us that if he would not gain weight within the next two weeks he would have to be hospitalized again.

At home, I fed him every two hours, just a tiny bit, just as much as he could take before taking his nap lying on my chest. As soon as he started waking up I fed him again, holding him while he was asleep until feeding time again. This went on day and night for the next two weeks. I was exhausted although my husband took over some of the evening "shifts." Most of the time we both napped together, then I fed him and we napped again. I held him close, told him stories of all the adventures that were waiting for him in this life and that he had to eat to grow strong, I rocked him and sang to him. Would I call all of this meditation, chanting, prayers—absolutely. It all came naturally back then, and it was my only comfort.

The day of the next visit to the doctor arrived, and I anxiously awaited the news. My intuition told me that all would be good, that my prayers had been heard. And so it was! He had gained just enough weight to keep him from being hospitalized. Energized and encouraged that all my efforts had worked I took him home again, happy and overjoyed with the determination to raise a healthy, happy, strong child (and boy, if you know my son now, did my prayers work!!!!)

We kept making progress and indeed by the end of his first year there was no difference between him and other children his age.

Life was good once again—for a little while anyways. My deep faith, belief in prayers and ability to go into deep meditation had saved my son and I am certain of that now, although had no idea what I was doing back then.

Soon, there was another challenge appearing on the horizon—after all, life is that way, right? How would we grow if not through challenges?

Our marriage started to deteriorate. My husband drank too much, lost his job, and we ran into money troubles. Sometimes there wasn't even enough money for me to buy food or formula for our son. We lived in a little town and there were no jobs for either one of us. My parents helped out with money, but they could only do so much. They suggested for us to move to Bonn, where they lived, so they would be able to help us more.

Back to Bonn we went so my parents could watch our son while we both worked. We found a nice little apartment and things seemed to settle down. Then my husband got homesick. He had never been away from his hometown and could not make new friends. He wanted all of us to go back. I refused, but he went anyway. Long story short, we got divorced and I raised our son by myself. But life was good: I made decent money, we had the beautiful apartment to ourselves, we went on little vacations. Yet, I missed a partner in my life.

The Love of My Life?

I joined different social groups to meet people and had my first experience with yoga, but it didn't quite resonate with me at that time. I was more interested in finding "the guy." My next husband turned out to be a neighbor of mine. He was married when we first met and I wasn't even romantically interested in him but liked him and his wife. The two of them, my son and I did things together, hiked, attended events, cooked together. It was a fun time. Then H. told me that his marriage wasn't going too well and his wife had an affair with someone else. We spent many long hours talking, and him venting. We developed a wonderful friendship that soon evolved into a romantic relationship.

Long story short, they got divorced, we got married and finally I felt at home. He was a wonderful husband; we felt we were soul mates and it reflected in our marriage and our life together.

We planned our first child together and I got pregnant. I loved my pregnancy…

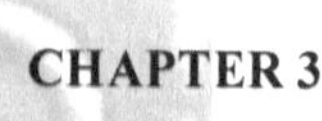

CHAPTER 3

How My Personal Yoga Journey Began

Then one day, during that pregnancy many years ago, I found a little green, very old book about yoga in a secondhand bookstore.

After discovering the old book about yoga, of course, at first, I was astonished and fascinated by the "contorted" positions the pictures showed. I started reading a little; the book was cheap, so I bought it and took it home. Then I began trying to copy the poses. Some poses were very easy (although now I realize I probably didn't do them right, missing the proper guidance of an experienced teacher), some very impossible, some were pleasant, others were a challenge. I kept reading and I kept doing the poses. I was intrigued, to say the least. I started setting aside a certain time of day for my yoga practice, and eagerly awaited that time. Of course, I had to be careful to practice the easier poses that were allowed during pregnancy. But I also found a book that demonstrated a woman from India who was doing ALL the poses throughout her entire pregnancy up until the day she gave birth (she had done yoga all her life, though, and had learned it from her father).

I was intrigued by learning about meditation and read as much as I could, and found a beautiful way to connect with my unborn baby through the stillness and concentration of meditation the same way I had done unknowingly with my first child.

All my pregnancies have been some of the most enjoyable times in my life. I literally glowed and radiated out love, compassion and total happiness.

Appreciation = The highest form of achieving, as Thich Nhat Hanh states, is "When you breathe in be aware of breathing in—when you breathe out be aware of breathing out."

Simple mindfulness in every moment of our lives can lead us to deep appreciation. Being appreciative for everything we encounter is so very important—there is a reason for it even if we don't see or understand it at the moment. Appreciate the people in your life, the lessons you learn through them, the gifts you receive through the blessing of their presence on your life path. Look around you and notice things as if it was the first time you see them. Appreciation leads to Gratitude to Joy to Happiness. SSP

And as much as I enjoyed this little life growing inside of me, I could hardly wait for the day to come to hold my baby.

It was Easter Monday when labor started and my water broke. We had just had a big meal with very garlicky leg of lamb, and even more garlic in the green beans. I was terrified at the thought of having to go to the hospital now after eating all that garlic. But there was no choice. When we got there they wanted me to take Valium and wait until Tuesday, as it was a holiday and I guess they didn't want to deliver. My husband and I were appalled; I took the Valium and threw it into the trash, not telling the nurses of course, and we let nature take its course as it was supposed to. Giving birth was easy. It only took two hours and K. was born. All the breathing techniques that I had learned were very similar to yogic breathing and helped tremendously. Everything went perfect, and with no complications, I had my son on my belly right away. He nursed a few moments later and we were given plenty of "getting to know each other" time.

What a difference to the experience of giving birth to his older brother six years ago, how much more we knew about bonding and the importance of the family staying together, having time to touch, and feel and smell. A happy family left the hospital a few hours later.

Happiness at home!!! Oh how we enjoyed our little boy. It was so much better to be in our own home rather than the hospital; especially after the experience the first time with my oldest son and not being able to hold him during those precious and important first hours, days and weeks.

All four of us lay in bed cuddling and admiring our newest "family member." Of course, this time I nursed and it was the most wonderful bonding experience possible that I so much missed to having with my oldest son.

From Happiness to Despair

Since we didn't stay in the hospital we had to go to the first checkup for K. on the third day. It was a devastating day. A heart murmur was discovered. He was scheduled immediately for a procedure to find out what exactly the issue was. Our hearts were racing along with our minds. Fear and desperation crept up in me. BREATHE—is all I could think. BREATHE—it will all be ok.

We took him home; I meditated while nursing my son. I kept him close in a baby sling, giving him love, health, strength twenty-four/seven. I knew that my love would get us through this. I had done it before with M., my oldest son, and it had to work again.

Not much time for the physical part of yoga anymore but meditation, yes, all the time.

Meditation—When I first started meditation practice many years ago I thought that by doing it all my conditions, suffering, and past hurts, would just go away and I simply would become centered and serene. Over time I realized that sitting means to sit still WITH all of it, allowing it to be as it is, accepting it and not needing to change anything about it. NO, I don't have to fix anything. What a relief! By just sitting with whatever it is, being present in this very moment and with consistency, simply accepting it overtime issues dissolve, burn up, strip away. Awareness is the answer, acceptance and sticking with our practice, turning this awareness inward. That way spaciousness is created as well as clarity, that in turn opens the door to compassion, first towards ourselves, then towards others. SSP

After the procedure was done, it was discovered that our baby boy had a huge ventricle septum defect (a large hole between the main chambers of the heart). We were told that he had a 50/50 chance to survive his first year, and that there was no surgery available at the time.

We were crushed, yet, my faith and belief and ability to meditate carried me through. I was determined that my little boy would live and thrive! I read everything I could get my hands on that dealt with alternative ways to feed him and I decided to nurse him for as long as possible, as that provided the best nutrition for him.

When he grew older of course I home-cooked his meals with all organic ingredients only. He was put on medication (digitalis) to help his heart function better. He learned to walk at nine months; he started talking at about the same time. His first birthday arrived and he seemed ok—what a celebration! I guarded him, enjoyed and cherished every second.

One day in deep meditation a thought came to me, almost a conviction—medicine advances all the time. What was a 50/50 chance yesterday could be an 80/50 next year, and a 100% a few years later. How true this proved itself. So here I had a goal, a hope, a dream: I had to do everything I could to keep him alive and well as long as possible. I knew there would be a way to fix his little heart. My part was to provide nourishment, love, faith, and determination that would give us time. And that is exactly what I did.

~

Feelings versus Emotions

Emotions are sensations in the body that can be triggered by memories, thoughts, and external stimuli, and they can change our physical state. Emotion has a "story" attached to it; there is a physical aspect as well as a psychological aspect; they control our thinking, behavior and actions.

The two basic emotions are love and fear. All other emotions, thoughts and behaviors are variations of these two. Anxiety, anger, control, sadness, depression, inadequacy, confusion, hurt, loneliness, guilt, shame—all of these are fear-based emotions. And joy, happiness, caring, trust, compassion, truth, contentment, satisfaction are love-based emotions.

A pure, not self-conscious state is considered a feeling.

We "feel" joy, for example, when we look at a baby, when we are absorbed in the moment, such as watching a beautiful sunset. A feeling is something more direct, something sensory sometimes. A feeling is something we can identify. SSP

Years went by; frequent check-ups confirmed that K. was still doing ok. He could not do all the things that kids his age were doing; he could not run, and even walking for a while exhausted him and his skin would turn bluish due to lack of oxygen. We bought him a mini ATV (very rare to come by in those years, especially in Germany). He was the hero on the playground, leaving everyone in the dust with his little vehicle. When we hiked we had to carry him on our backs for most of the time or pulled him in his little cart. We enjoyed it and got used to it. We accepted what was given to us. We would get through this. I just knew!

TRUTH AND RESISTANCE

When we reject feelings we reject parts of ourselves. These suppressed feelings will manipulate our future experiences.

When we do something we don't want to do, we are denying ourselves, which drains our energy and can cause sicknesses.

But if we don't open up to share our feelings, this is equally unhealthy.

Accepting our feelings—good or bad—and if necessary, working through them via expression, can allow the essence of our transformation and increase joy, unconditional love, sensuality, gratitude and forgiveness. SSP

CHAPTER 4

Through these years I picked up my regular physical yoga practice again, as well as continuing my regular meditation. Meditation sometimes was difficult as the fear of the future kept creeping in, but combining the yoga postures with the meditation and controlled breathing oftentimes did the trick, keeping my mind occupied and giving me peace and an hour or so to relax in my own little world. This allowed me to nurture myself and gain my strength back, to be the support that I needed to be for my family.

Keeping my Faith

Then another fate struck us. My husband was diagnosed with testicular cancer. I remember how I sat on the couch and cried my eyes out; how would we survive? Surgery had to come first, then months of radiation and chemo, would he die? How would I live with my two sons and no formal education?

I turned to my inner wisdom once more. I trusted my intuition and my faith yet again. Surgery was immediately necessary, so we did it. It was no big deal…but the months of chemo were. My husband was a hero—he kept his pain and misery mostly from me and the kids, but sometimes when on a trip, we had to stop and he had to throw up. He was exhausted, working all the time while undergoing treatment.

I prayed, I meditated, I found strength. I researched alternative ways of treatment. I studied **holistic medicine** just for the purpose of keeping my husband alive. Here I was, struggling along with a child with a severe heart defect and a husband with cancer. I was the only one who was able to stay strong and it was my obligation too. There was no time for me to be afraid.

WHEN FEAR KNOCKS ON THE DOOR…and love answers—nobody's there.

Fear is a powerful feeling, disguising itself in many forms such as feeling nothing, rage, hopelessness, feeling numb. How does fear control our lives? Holding back out of fear of rejection?

Letting people walk all over us out of fear of not being accepted? Taking on more than we can handle out of fear to appear not capable? Doing things we don't want to do out of fear of not being loved?

The list goes on. What are we so afraid of? Learning to express our true feelings will bring healing and expanded awareness; we will experience a higher plane of consciousness.

Letting go of ego, being kind rather than being right, loving ourselves just the way we are because we are the result of divine creation will send fear packing and leave and it will open the door wide to let love into our lives. Where love reigns—fear cannot enter. SSP

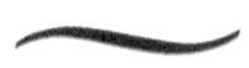

We completely changed our diet to organic and mostly vegetarian. I researched specific supplements, and interviewed alternative practitioners (something almost unheard of back in those days). I learned a lot and we experimented. My husband got better, but there it was again—that looming fear of death. I was confronted with the thought of death on a daily basis for the last five years at least, not only for my sons but now also about my husband. But then, death is a natural part of life, isn't it?

~

Reflection—*It is primarily through our resistances, difficulties, challenges, problems, illnesses, etc. that we eventually begin to discover what they are for and why they exist. Delving deeply enough into the energy behind them leads us to sufficiently overcome some ignorance, selfishness and inertia, allowing us to get glimpses of the beautiful soul energy causing them. Taking this journey to our essence and to our purpose eventually shifts our conscious identity to the soul that we are. Look behind the appearance of something in your life that you have not welcomed or understood, and discover more deeply who you really are. SSP*

~

Time went by. My husband completely recovered but we had been told that we would not be able to have any more children due to the radiation and chemo. As much as I had wanted more children, especially a little girl after my two boys, I was ok with it. It was more important that my husband was well and had recovered.

Life went almost back to normal. Another few years went by, K. was still doing ok. My heart was full of gratitude for those seven years that I had with him already despite the devastating diagnosis at his birth.

The one who probably suffered the most though all of this was my oldest son: he was neglected because all the attention went to his sick little brother first then to his sick step dad and back to his little brother. And yet he watched him and played with him and protected him wherever he could. I did not see what lay under the surface. A wounded little boy, just as I had experienced in my own childhood. He failed in school, got himself into all kinds of trouble, he was challenged at home and did not receive the support and nurturing that a little boy needs. I could see all this years later but at that time I was overwhelmed myself. My heart aches and my soul cries thinking back to what he must have endured and gone through. Unfortunately, I did not realize it at that time.

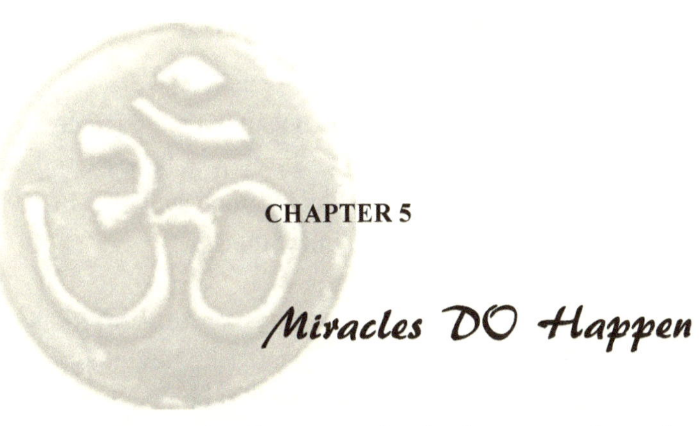

CHAPTER 5

Miracles DO Happen

Just when my family was getting back to normal, another miracle happened. I went to my yearly physical checkup, and after all the tests the doctor inquired if there might be a chance I may be pregnant. I told him that I had not had my period for about three months, but that we were told that I could not get pregnant because of my husband's earlier illness and treatment. A quick test revealed indeed I WAS PREGNANT. I could not believe it; I thought it must have been a mistake. Another test, ultrasound, there was no question! Joy!!! Overjoyed!!!

Joy

Your purpose in life is the expression of soul qualities, which bring joy and happiness. When you are doing something that you think you should be doing as part of your life's purpose and you do not feel joy in it, or it does not take you out of your personality, then you have to question if this is what you ought to be doing. Reflect on something you are doing in your life and ask yourself if it really is aligned with what is most appropriate for you?

Life had another new purpose! Another dream came true. Another miracle happened. So I was four months pregnant and hadn't had a clue. I was walking on clouds. However, we were told that we should have an amniocentesis to make sure the baby was ok due to our son's heart defect possibly running in the family, and the radiation and chemo that my husband had received. We agreed, although I made it clear that abortion was not an option, no matter what the outcome of the test would be. I was ready to have a child that was disabled as well as a healthy child. I would have this baby, no matter what. And, I also wanted to know the sex!

The result was overwhelming, not only was my baby ok from what they could tell but I was expecting a little GIRL!!! Now the fun really began: pink, pink, everywhere, I bought pink baby clothes and bedding, pink outfits for myself, even pink glasses; but most of all I delved again into deep meditation, this time with lots of thoughts of gratitude, deep reverence for life and the appreciation of my faith. Again and again these virtues had been the source of tremendous strength in my life and would continue to do so.

Finally—Yoga Again!

I picked up my gentle yoga practice again. I knew how important this aspect of my life has always been, and the time was right to immerse myself into yoga practice again wholeheartedly, body, mind and spirit.

Everybody knows the story about when one is pregnant and all one sees is pregnant women everywhere, now that happened to me with yoga. Suddenly I saw certain ads in the paper about yoga AND best of all there was a yoga class offered in my little town where I lived at that time. No question that I would sign up for it.

I could hardly wait for the day to come for my first yoga class. My husband even agreed to come home earlier from work to take care of the kids so I could go. I was sooo excited, but also a little nervous. What if all the others would be more flexible than I? What if I couldn't do certain things? What if I made a fool of myself after all this time not being too physically active?

The moment the instructor walked in, all my worries disappeared. She was probably in her fifties, so no competition for me, in my thirties then—or so I thought. All the other women were about my age as well, so I felt pretty good. She was an inspiration from the first moment on. I wanted to be like her. She had this aura of calm, strength, goodness. In her fifties she was as flexible as a willow tree, she flowed through the poses with grace and ease compared to all of us who were so much younger. But she did not show off, instead she was kind and encouraging.

"What then is it this joy of manifesting from allowing that makes me want so much to be a better allower? At the end of a hard working day, or better yet, a softly woven day what can one say to the things that accumulated around; 'Goodnight sweet light, see you in the morning dear bed, sleep tight big TV set, or I love you closet of clothes.' No, it is not things that bring living-joy; it is the appreciation of these desired manifestations that enlighten-up the space between having and applying, owning and using, wanting and getting." The Art of Appreciation, by Peggy Halevi

It turned out my instructor was absolutely wonderful, not only caring, kind, gentle AND strong, but also flexible as well as tough. She was exactly how a good instructor should be. She gently guided us through some breathing exercises, explaining the importance of the breath as the initiator for the movement (never the other way around). We learned that through the gentle control of the breath our minds could be controlled and stilled to prepare us for deeper meditation. We learned some simple yoga asanas (postures) such as a gentle forward fold (standing as well as sitting on the floor), some gentle twists and backbends. At the end of the class we were guided through **Savasana** (corpse pose, relaxation at the end of each yoga class), needless to say that I felt fabulous after this first class! In fact, this was really one of my first serious yoga classes. My previous practice had been at home based on books, which I absolutely do not recommend with the knowledge that I now have as a yoga instructor.

So I continued my weekly yoga classes with my instructor and practiced at home as well. Of course, I talked to my instructor about the pregnancy, and she assured me that after all my practice by that time it would be fine for me to continue with a few adaptations. I was relieved, as I could not imagine my life without my yoga practice anymore. The benefits were tremendous. Through the practice of alignment and proper movement I had none of some of the common ailments associated with being pregnant. Not only did I not have any morning sickness (although I didn't have that with my first two pregnancies either), I had no backaches or breathing problems—what a relief!

I kept my practice up until about three weeks before the due date. By that time, I just was too big and heavy. Now was the time I consciously used meditation more and more, connecting on a very special level with my little girl.

The Miraculous Power of Yoga

The day came when we had to go to the hospital. I was excited and prepared, refusing any medication as I was determined to have a natural birth. It took long, very long, two days of labor, no progress, and it turned out she lay sideways. I was exhausted, tired, disheartened. The doctors suggested a C-section. I was even more disappointed. The doctors and nurses left to make preparations for the procedure and my husband and I were alone for a few moments. He was trying to cheer me up and mentioned that "certain yoga pose where Mira always woke up." I smiled and went into "happy baby pose" and instantly she turned around and into the right position, we both could see it actually happening, and of course I felt it. Then everything happened so fast. The doctors and nurses came back into the room, and all I heard them saying was "oh my god I can see her black hair already?" It took a few more moments and our miracle baby was born. Did I mention that yoga has worked many many miracles in my life??

Our little girl was named Mira—the miracle baby.

Miracles

Mira was healthy and the calmest of all my three children. She slept through the night from the second day on. She slept most of the day. I nursed her of course, and did the same meditation practice while breast-feeding her as I had done with K. We did little gentle yoga moves together. Life was good again.

The Power of Prayer

Then another checkup came up for K. and we were told that the medicine was no longer working and he would need surgery soon. The good news was that there was a procedure available now that had a very high success rate—my prayers and faith had worked.

PART 2

Hatred can never cease by hatred.
Hatred can only cease by love.
This is an eternal law.

~ The Buddha

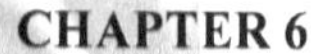

CHAPTER 6

The Dreaded Day Turns into a New Life

Once the surgery was scheduled, we were told it would take about eight hours and that it would be best if we went home to wait. Since we had the two other children, we chose to go home.

I retreated into my meditation space immediately; I started with deep breathing to calm my racing mind and was able to go into deep meditation fairly quickly. It was more of a continuous prayer than a meditation. I visualized the perfect outcome, I visualized my little boy surrounded and protected by angels. I had this tremendous faith and belief that all would be good. About two hours into my "retreat," somebody knocked on the door. I was startled. It was my husband. The hospital had just called; in fact they were still on the line to get our permission for a different kind of surgery. Our son was laying on the operating table, cut open, on life-support while they were talking to us. I freaked for a moment, but the next second I calmed down. I knew this was the solution I had been praying for. We quickly got the scope on why and what type of surgery. And as I had prayed and hoped, there was a better option for our son that would promise a much more desirable outcome. Of course we decided fast and gave our permission to go ahead.

I went back into my meditation, this time even more sure of the perfect outcome. Maybe I even had an "out of body" experience as I felt very close to my little boy. I was holding his hand, softly singing to him, telling him to hang on and that all would be ok.

I always know exactly when to come out of meditation and when that happened I knew that everything was complete, done, perfect.

Emotions were running high for the entire family, even the grandparents, and I honestly don't even remember what happened in between. It must have been at least a day later because when we got to ICU K. was awake. Everybody cried to see his little body bruised, bandaged and so fragile and PALE—but I smiled, for the first time in his entire life his skin was NOT BLUE—he was just pale, as everybody would be after an invasive procedure like that. It meant that his blood got enough oxygen and that the surgery must have been successful. I never knew before that what the word "relief" could mean.

Needless to say, I followed up and ended the day with more meditation. Gratitude.

~

Limitlessness

I am bathed in an ocean of gratitude and guidance

As I begin my journey out from the center

I surrender to the next step

Which carries me toward

My natural state of limitlessness,

Inner completeness,

As I now prepare for my dharmic path of learning. SSP

~

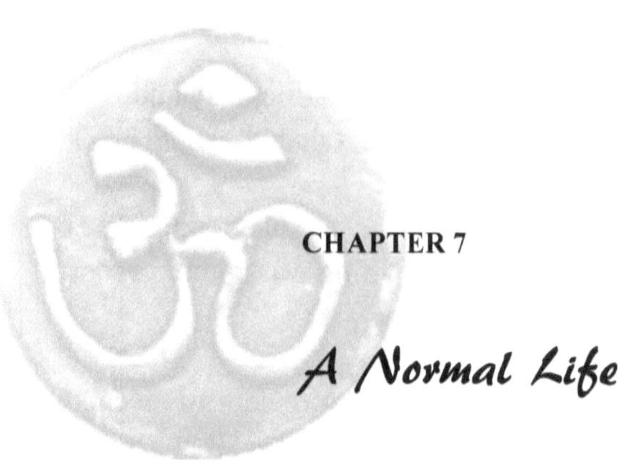

CHAPTER 7

A Normal Life

K. only had to stay in the hospital for three weeks and then we were able to take him home. A little anxiety crept up since the surgery took place at sea level in a different part of Germany, yet our home at that time was in Bavaria at about 800 meters elevation. We watched him closely; constant and regular checkups were necessary, but all was good and there seemed to be no complications.

I was finally able to completely relax.

A time of happiness and peace came into my life. My kids went to school/kindergarden in the morning, giving me plenty of time to eventually take care of myself.

I kept my morning meditation practice up, followed by the physical yoga practice. I enjoyed the peace and quiet and having the house to myself for a few hours. Several years went by without any major challenges for our family; it was a time we all needed to recover from all the stresses of the previous years.

We all loved Bavaria and the little village we lived in. We took fabulous hikes in the mountains of Bavaria, Austria, Switzerland and K. was doing just fine. We went to Italy, Spain, France—we were just a normal family and it felt so good.

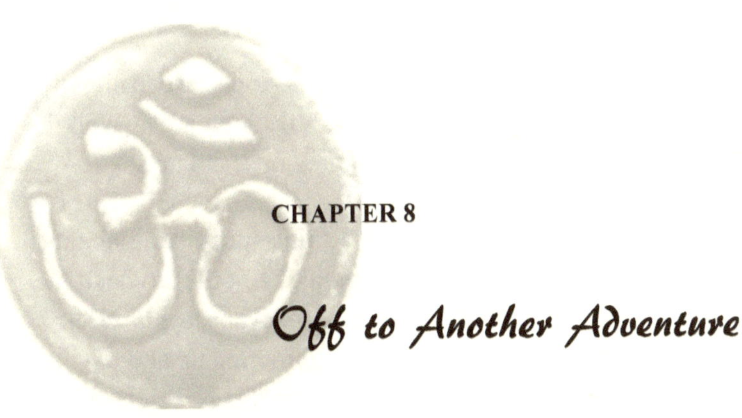

CHAPTER 8

Off to Another Adventure

With the family stable and all of our nerves relaxed, an adventure was presented to us—a South American adventure. Yes, that's right. After several years of living without challenges I guess we needed one again. My husband got a job offer in South America. But this was a journey I was up for, and, of course, so was he. We went for a "test" trip to Bogota/Colombia, out of all places.

I don't blame the reader for thinking that we were crazy, but yes, we did just that—moved to the drug capital of the world.

It was a tremendous job opportunity for my husband and we thought it would also be a once in a lifetime chance to explore and experience a totally different country, not only on a vacation, but to actually live there. The decision was made and preparations taken. How exciting!

We rented a—what at first sight seemed to be—beautiful Spanish style villa in a conjunto (a guarded community, fenced for security) surrounded by avocado, citrus, and palm trees. The first few weeks went by in a flash: the kids were put into a private upscale Swiss school, we joined an exclusive country club, and drove expensive cars. We were invited to elegant upper management parties; I had my personal tailor to make all the fancy dresses necessary to show off at those parties. I took tennis and riding lessons at the club with the kids. We took trips to the Caribbean and into the

Colombian jungle, as well as high up into the Andes. I can already envision the reader thinking, "and this is still Sophia???" Well, it really wasn't my kind of lifestyle, but more on that later.

When I got sick the first time, I didn't think much of it, as that was fairly common in a third world country. But the stomach flu kept coming back to a point where out of seven days a week I spent at least five hanging over the toilet, throwing up and having diarrhea. After several months I had lost so much weight that I had no strength left to do anything. I was diagnosed with Giardia among other things. I was put on drugs that would eventually destroy my liver and immune system.

It was time to consult my good old friend—meditation. Since there wasn't much else for me to do—I had a "muchacha" (cleaning lady), a driver, gardener and anything else one would dream of. I was too weak to go horseback riding or to play tennis, so I had plenty of time to meditate. As usual, a sense of peace and acceptance came over me in this deep state of relaxation. I had nobody to blame for this—I was as much a part of the decision to come to this country as anybody else. I had better find a way to deal with it.

Water wisdom

"When flowing water . . . meets with obstacles on its path, a blockage in its journey, it pauses. It increases in volume and strength, filling up in front of the obstacle and eventually spilling past it . . . .

"Do not turn and run, for there is nowhere worthwhile for you to go. Do not attempt to push ahead into the danger . . . emulate the example of the water: Pause and build up your strength until the obstacle no longer represents a blockage."

—from the 'I Ching,'

However, I also knew that I needed proper treatment and a clean environment to gain my strength back. We had friends in California and they invited us to visit for Christmas, which would be a relief for me to feel as though I was in a clean safe country. In California, I could practically eat anything and not get sick. Whereas in Colombia—the land of fresh tropical fruit and vegetables and fresh juices—I had to revert to "dead" cooked meats and vegetables to make sure that all the germs were gone. What a shame that, despite the exotic beauty of this tropical country, my body thought otherwise.

My husband and I decided to look for a vacation home in California so we had a safe place to come to and for me to recover. He went back to Colombia for work and I stayed with our daughter. We spent two weeks with realtors but could not find anything that would fit our budget since what we really wanted was a house at the beach (for about 200k—dream on!)

Disillusioned and disheartened, my daughter and I flew back to Bogota.

The path to wholeness

We think that God has blessed us if we don't have too many troubles. In fact, religions have erroneously taught us that pain is punishment for our sins. We often ask, "What have I done wrong?" when things do not go the way we want.

Yet, to become ourselves in the truest and deepest sense, we must face our own duality, which of course includes facing our darkness. As souls we strive for wholeness, not for perfection.

At first, we really don't know what is going on. We just find life difficult, challenging and often painful. Eventually, after much experience and reflection, we start to find meaning in it all. Eventually, we gladly accept the means whereby we can do the Soul work we have come for.

As we become conscious as Souls, we walk our journey purposefully, embracing the reality of our earthly nature along with the truth of our divine nature.

"When we are conscious of our personal uniqueness and our universal nature we express ourselves creatively. In this way we fulfill our dreams and our life purpose."

—Andrew Schneider

CHAPTER 9

The Start of Something Big

Once we returned to South America, I unpacked the suitcases with all the goodies we had brought back from the U.S., and at the bottom I found my shoes wrapped in some newspaper. At that time, I cherished anything that had to do with NORTH America (actually I still do as it is the country of my dreams) so I straightened the paper out and glanced at it. An advertisement from a Real Estate Company popped out and caught my eye.

Those who know me know how my intuition kicks in and I spring into action. That is exactly what I did. I typed up a letter (I did not have email at that time) that we were looking for a vacation home in the U.S. and then faxed it out "into the world." Only a few days later I received a call from the agent, Kathy, asking me where we wanted a vacation home. I told her that our preference was California, and she informed me that she was an agent in Colorado. My answer was, "where the heck is Colorado?" She explained the geography of the region to me, adding that the Rocky Mountains snaked right through the middle. She spoke of wide, open spaces, vast forests, wildlife, clean air, good roads . . . . I could see it all in my mind's eye. She assured me that we could easily find a place for less than 200k.

That same night, my husband and I made the decision that I would fly to Colorado to find us a vacation home.

The realtor promised she would arrange for my arrival and pick me up at the airport. On top of that, she insisted I stay with her and her husband at their apartment in downtown Denver so she would take care of me.

I was sad to leave my family behind but I was also very excited about this "new challenge" for me (I think that is just my fate, that I keep needing new challenges).

I boarded the plane. It was only a six-hour-flight, straight up north basically. I couldn't wait to get there. We were about to land when I thought I was going to die. The plane bounced up and down and I heard a terrible screeching noise. Then the plane stopped and I was still alive. We were informed that a tire blew while landing. Welcome to the United States of America!

CHAPTER 10

America

Upon arrival, I thanked the heavens I had my German passport as I was directed to another line (the one for the "safe countries" I guess) and went through customs in no time, where my poor Colombian fellow travelers were still being questioned and interrogated.

There was Kathy and her husband Jim; friendly, welcoming people, just what Americans are. Jim took my luggage and they steered me through the busy airport. I couldn't believe my eyes—they picked me up in a huge limousine. I felt like a movie star.

Looking out the window on the drive to downtown Denver I was expecting to see the Rocky Mountains, but all I saw were those little hills. Disappointed, I asked Kathy if those were the mountains I wished to see. "Oh no," she replied, "These are just the foothills. The Rockies are in the clouds today. You will see them tomorrow!"

Their downtown apartment was huge with windows on all sides; I could see the skyscrapers as well as the Rockies the next morning. I had a beautiful guest room with mountain views. It was perfect for my familiar practice. No yoga mat; a towel on the floor would have to do. Oh how I cherished the gentle moves to stretch out my body after the flight, the deep breathing and meditation to calm me down after all the excitement.

The next morning we had our pow-wow. I needed to establish a bank account and credit before we even could get started on the real estate part.

We got that done by ten that morning, then went to Kathy's office. She searched for properties, set showings and off we went. The first few were condos in Golden—not what I had visualized.

I wanted a cabin in the woods, in the mountains with a little land. First it seemed there was nothing like that out there, but then she found a property in Bailey, it was in the last stages of being finished, so I could easily choose all the personalized décor like bathroom tiles, carpet and paint color.

Off we went again. Highway 285 for the first time! All I could see was the highway, mountains, and forests. I knew THIS was more what I was looking for. We took the exit and came to our destination, a subdivision called "Friendship Ranch." What an inviting name! It sounded like home already. We drove up to the property, and I immediately knew that this was it! Three bedrooms, two baths, large open kitchen/living space and a den, garage with a deck as big as a ballroom (overstated, but that's what it felt like to me), brand new, not even finished yet, surrounded by tall spruce trees, Ponderosa pine and aspens.

I called my husband as soon as we got back to town and we wrote the offer. Finances were not an issue as we had good credit. The offer was accepted, and closing was set for mid-May. Now what?

The gift of joy

Allow the dust and grit of the past become the compost and nurturing for the blossoming, growing and thriving of your true self. Let go of all doubt, fear and feeling of inadequacy and invite joy, trust, love and the awareness of the present moment to manifest in you. Once we manifested those qualities in ourselves we can radiate them out to others.

Joy is one of the greatest gifts we can give to people around us. Those who are unhappy need our joy, not our sadness.   SSP

"Joy is prayer—Joy is strength—Joy is love—Joy is a net of love by which you can catch souls. She gives most who gives with Joy."

—Mother Teresa

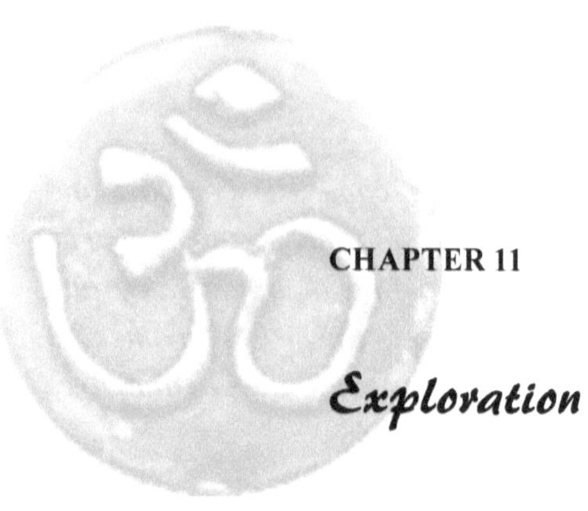

CHAPTER 11

Exploration

After all the paperwork, I had the chore and obligation to stay until closing! Since there wasn't much for me to do I decided to take a trip to Taos, New Mexico. I felt on top of the world, as it was the first trip I had taken by myself since I got married and had children; I almost felt guilty but at the same time decided to enjoy every second of it. The drive was beautiful and whoever took that same route knows what I am talking about. Up Highway 285 towards Kenosha Pass/South Park, the wide open expanse of meadows and forests, the distant snowcapped mountains, deer and elk on the side of the road. This was like a safari, only better.

A profound sense of gratitude settled deep into my heart. Gradually, a feeling of belonging grew stronger and stronger inside of me. I looked at the deep blue Colorado sky as if I had never seen the sky before and I knew there were no limits in what I could do. By looking at this vast expanse of trees I realized that I would grow roots here, and the mountains instilled the possibility of stability, safety and trust deep into my soul.

Is it possible to meditate while driving? It depends on how we define meditation: if I am totally present and mindfully in the moment—which I was—then yes, it is possible (and I am not suggesting to the reader to close their eyes and withdraw their senses). Every second was fully appreciated, fully lived, fully experienced. Every mile I drove that day was pure wonder, reverence and gratefulness. I rolled down the windows to experience every deep breath of fresh, cool, crisp, clean mountain air—it was as if I was breathing for the first time in my life.

Look to this day, for it is life, the very life of life. In its brief course lie all the realities and verities of existence. The bliss of growth, the splendor of action, the glory of power. And yesterday is but a dream, and tomorrow is only a vision. But today—well lived—makes every yesterday a dream of happiness, and every tomorrow a vision of hope. Look well, therefore, to this day.~ Sanskrit proverb ~

There were no thoughts of yesterday or tomorrow, just this very moment was what mattered. I knew that I had arrived; although in the true sense I felt that I had embarked on an important journey, and that this journey was more important than the destination.

Although, I knew that the cabin wasn't yet ours, and I had to go back to my family in South America, and that I would get sick again—but deep down in my heart it also was clear to me that there was something big and profound growing, evolving and surrounding me; something that would change my life forever.

"When you are inspired by some great purpose, some extraordinary project, all your thoughts break their bonds; your mind transcends limitations, your consciousness expands in every direction, and you find yourself in a new, great and wonderful world. Dormant forces, faculties and talents come alive, and you discover yourself to be a greater person by far than you ever dreamed yourself to be."—Patanjali

CHAPTER 12

Starting a New Life?

My visit to New Mexico was fabulous. I stayed in a beautiful bed and breakfast, had great food and shopped. The days flew by and it was time to drive back to Denver. By that time, I decided to find a hotel rather than enjoying Jim and Kathy's hospitality. They did not want to let me go but I felt that I needed to give them back their privacy. Plus, it would only be a few more weeks until closing.

I started buying household items for the new cabin and "stacked" them in the hotel room. Every day I drove up to the mountains to our cabin, talked with the construction crew, made decisions on the tile, carpet, wall colors. When they all left at 5 pm, I stayed and "bonded" with the new place. The cabin was open and spacious with large windows, allowing the warm Colorado sun to spill indoors. I sat on the deck, watching deer and foxes while slowly drifting off into meditations. My heart was filled with wonder and gratitude for the miracles that were happening in my life. It was May and the days were long already. I usually stayed until the sun went down, and then drove back to town.

The day of the closing came, and I remember when I finally got the keys to our cabin. The rented SUV was loaded to the brim with all the furniture, kitchen items, bedding, and all I would need in my mountain retreat, for a few days at least.

It was probably one of the happiest moments in my life when I opened the door to the cabin that day. A dream had come true and the cabin was ours. In no time I had turned almost every room into something resembling "my" space.

Time to roll out the yoga mat on the deck. Every breath I took, every yoga move I made was a prayer of gratitude.

I had never done yoga on a deck, let alone under towering pine trees. Everything felt so right, so perfect.

"Be willing to allow much and much will arrive. Appreciate and more things to appreciate come into your life." The Art of Appreciation, by Peggy Halevi

I spent the evenings on the deck as well, watching the stars appear one by one in the midnight blue sky. The sky in the city with its reflecting lights mostly hid the stars from sight, but not here. No city lights, the next-door neighbor far enough away, there was nothing to disturb the sacredness of this moment. The air got cool and crisp, I wrapped myself in a blanket; I just could not go inside yet. Many shooting stars crossed the sky, some quick, some in a long beautiful arc that would have allowed for many wishes. But instead of making wishes I sent gratitude out with every one that appeared and disappeared.

The next morning I heard a roaring sound and was wondering what it was—the wind in the towering pine trees. What a powerful song these ancient giants were singing for me. Standing barefoot on the deck in my pajamas something caught my eye, just a quick movement. A herd of deer was grazing in the front yard, just a few feet from me. I could hardly believe what I saw; they did not seem to be afraid, just looking at me. Never in my life had I been this close to wildlife, let alone in a totally natural setting.

My three days at the cabin went by in a flash—time to get back to my family in South America.

"Today I will witness the choices I make in each moment. And in the mere witnessing of these choices, I will bring them to my conscious awareness. I will know that the best way to prepare for any moment in the future is to be fully conscious in the present. Whenever I make a choice, I will ask myself two questions: "What are the consequences of this choice that I'm making?" and "Will this choice bring fulfillment and happiness to me and also to those who are affected by this choice?" I will then ask my heart for guidance and be guided by its message of comfort or discomfort. (Deepak Chopra)

CHAPTER 13

New Developments

Back in Colombia I could not speak the words as fast as I wanted to about all the wonders I had experienced in our new place. I was overflowing with excitement, stories and happiness.

Our plan was for all of us to spend the summer in Bailey. What an adventure to look forward to.

Time flew with preparation for the trip, and the day of the departure came.

Six hours later, there we were at Denver International Airport, and two hours after that we finally arrived at our cabin in the woods. My family loved it as much as I did. We went shopping to finish the furnishing, explored the neighborhood including all the fabulous hiking trails, creeks and rivers, then embarked on a spectacular trip to Yellowstone National Park. None of us had ever seen anything like that; buffalo, bears, moose, elk, wolves. Of course we visited Old Faithful and the geysers throughout the park, as well. The entire trip was like a fairy tale.

However, we were drawn back home to the cabin. Six weeks passed quickly and it was time to go to Colombia again. Nobody wanted to leave. I cried. How could I possibly leave paradise? We promised each other to come back for Christmas.

Life was not the same for any one of us after that summer, having experienced the wide-open space, clean air and environment, and wildlife. It was not easy to live in a polluted city with crime so horrible, I want to spare the reader the details. All that matters was getting through the days until Christmas and going "back home to the cabin."

Then some dramatic events occurred that changed our plans. First, we had a 6.9 earthquake, which immobilized Bogota for several days. Luckily, our house was old and built solidly out of rock and it was only a two-story, so there was not much damage. This was not so in the high-rise buildings downtown or the newer apartment buildings. Cell phones did not work. I had no idea if anything had happened to my husband who worked in downtown Bogota. My children's school was just across from our "conjunto," so I ran to get them. They were safe and all gathered on the lawns around the school. I took them home, just grateful that we all survived.

A few weeks after that, a friend of ours was killed by guerilla. They faked a minor accident to make him stop and get out of the car; he was trained (as all overseas companies train their employees and their family members) what to do in such a case and he did all the right things; he offered his wallet, watch, car; they took it all AND shot him.

Shortly after that in approximately the same area I was driving when I noticed in the rear view mirror a car driving erratically, it appeared as if he wanted to purposefully hit my car. It took me only seconds to realize that it was the same scenario that had happened to our friend who got murdered. There was no time for me to freak out. It all happened so quickly. I was the first one at the traffic light that had just turned red—I sped up, ignoring the red light and speeding across the intersection, merely avoiding being hit by other traffic. But I made it—the car that tried to hit me didn't.

That night my husband and I had a serious conversation. We decided that the children and I would remain in the U.S. after our Christmas vacation. He would go back to his work in Bogota, but we would try to find him another job in a safer country.

CHAPTER 14

Finding a Sanctuary

Somehow we made it thought those last weeks in Colombia, only because of the anticipation of our wonderful time to come in Colorado.

It probably was the most magnificent Christmas that we had ever had in our family. Here we were in our cozy cabin, Colorado champagne snow falling, with quiet, solitude, safety and peace.

We still needed to find a solution for our planned exit from Colombia. Up to that time we used our Visitor's Visa but that would only grant us three months of stay.

We consulted with an attorney; there were not very many options for us. The only one, and most appealing, was for me to get a Student Visa and go to school in order keep our legal status.

This was something I had been thinking about for a while. I wanted to have job again doing something meaningful. What an opportunity! Once again: out of sheer desperation and chaos came order.

What would I do? What would I study? I had not given it much thought until then. When I walked into the lobby of Red Rocks Community College the first flyer I saw was the announcement for a Park Ranger class. That's it—I love nature, to be in it, to protect it, to observe it. I met with the international student advisor; I enrolled within minutes. Mission accomplished. Practicing "the art of allowing" by being open and receptive to whatever comes our way had once again proved to be the best thing to do. I was thrown into a situation, I had no specific expectation other than making all this work for our family and the perfect opportunity presented itself to me; another turning point in my life. To me, that was evidence once again that the universe always provides exactly what we need, when we need it.

Visa problems settled, me now being a student Colorado REALLY felt like home, and I was determined to continue on this path of being open, receptive and allowing. Being a student was a completely new concept for me, but I thoroughly enjoyed it. It was the perfect course of study, being in Colorado's great outdoors. I learned all about wilderness survival, maps and following a compass, along with backcountry travel and hiking. I got so involved that I even joined the Colorado Mountain Club, took classes in backpacking/camping, participated in a leadership class and went on many hikes and backpacking trips before becoming a trip leader myself. This was something I had never done in my life and I felt exhilarated. I started climbing Fourteeners. I discovered how hiking, walking, and climbing could turn into a meditation; matching each step to the breath, taking in nature's beauty with great appreciation, physically moving beyond what I thought my body was capable of doing. I had found my place and loved my classes.

The kids went to a local school and I was able to schedule my classes so that I still was home when they were home for the most part.

I was looking forward to my birthday in our new home. My husband had promised to visit, as our birthdays were only a week apart. A few days before he called telling us that he couldn't make it because of his busy work schedule, which was a big disappointment but we knew he would come for vacation in summer. Weeks went by, the summer went by, but he did not come, giving one excuse after another. My daughter's birthday came in September and dad did not come. I knew something was not right, but I could not pinpoint it, and my husband assured us that he was just busy. No visit on Thanksgiving, but the promise that for sure he would be home for Christmas.

I started wondering, am I going to get divorced?

Early in the morning two days before Christmas came THE call from my husband. He would not come, he had met another woman, he did not love me anymore and wanted to marry her instead. I heard his voice as through a thick fog, but I could not say a word, just hung up. What would I say to our children?

Both of them came down to my bedroom and sat on the bed with me. They must have known from the look on my face that something terrible had just happened and I simply told them what he had told me. We all sat there, hugging each other, crying. My mind was blank. I felt paralyzed. I knew I had to do something, but what?

As usual I needed the solitude and comfort of nature. I needed to be alone to figure it all out. I know my kids were afraid I would leave them too, but I assured them that I just had to go for a walk to clear my head, and that I would be back soon. I went to one of my favorite hiking trails, the Kenosha part of the Colorado trail, where a section of huge, tall aspen trees always made me feel like being in a cathedral. I put my snowshoes on and headed up the snowy trail. I still could not think of a solution and suddenly the tears came. I stopped in my "cathedral," sobbing, tears streaming down my face. I felt completely lost, alone, discarded. Time did not exist at that moment and it did not matter. I just stood there motionless, without any feelings or thoughts or plans. Suddenly it felt as if there was a presence of something very comforting, almost as if someone was wrapping arms around me. It was so real that I turned around, but of course there was nobody there. I felt warm and protected and I heard a kind, gentle voice telling me that all would be okay, that I should go home to my children and that this was the Divine plan for my life, and that one day I would understand. To this day I don't know what happened, but I know that what I had heard and witnessed was the truth. I had to keep my faith and trust that things would work out just fine. So many times in my life I had been in situations that seemed hopeless, but by returning to my own center and keeping my faith and trust it always worked out. I turned around and drove home to comfort my kids.

We made it through Christmas as best as we could and it was quiet, peaceful and beautiful, just because we were together and assured each other that we would make it through this. Cuddling together under the tree, holding each other—isn't that what Christmas is really about?

CHAPTER 15

Support

Go Forward With Courage. When you are in doubt, be still, and wait; when doubt no longer exists for you, then go forward with courage. . . .So long as mists envelop you, be still; be still until the sunlight pours through and dispels the mists—as it surely will. Then act with courage. White Eagle

I realized that playtime was over and I better get an education and a degree in order to support my family. As a park ranger I would not make enough money, so I enrolled in an Associates program for Multimedia and Graphic Design. This had also been a dream and talent of mine since I was a child; I loved to work with colors, shapes, draw, create. I was probably the oldest student in the class, nevertheless I aced it and got my degree with a 4.0 GPA before securing a fabulous job as a Graphic Designer in a Travel Journal company. The downside was that I had to drive to town every day, leaving at 6 am and returning home at 7 pm; but my children matured quickly and took over many household chores. K. took over the role of "the man in the house" fixing things, doing yard work, and M. cooked, cleaned, did laundry. We were a happy family, and well-functioning for that matter, despite all of our challenges.

The divorce was a different matter. Because my husband and I are both German, it was difficult for me to find an attorney since

I was living in the U.S. with our children and he (by now) in a European country. All in all the divorce stretched out over five years, and it was a nightmare.

Being Open to Change

While I loved my job, all the driving took a toll on me and I kept thinking about something that I could do from home. That's when I discovered a Holistic Health program at the nearest community college. At first I was more interested in the classes for my own healing from the trauma of the divorce, but then I realized that there was some potential of a different kind of career for me as the program offered a certification upon completing it. I took every class offered and got my certificate.

At the same time I enrolled in a program for a degree as a Doctor of Naturopathy; half way through that I joined a yoga teacher program. Everything was coming together. I had no intention of becoming a yoga teacher, but wanted to advance my own yoga practice, which had suffered some by me being so busy in my life. It was a tough program—four days a week for six months—but I loved it. At the end during our final exam my instructor told me that I would never be a good yoga teacher; apparently my teaching was not coming from my heart. Although I never wanted to be a yoga teacher in the first place, her comment crushed me. I thought of myself as a loving, compassionate person whose delight was in helping others to advance; so why had she just told me the opposite?

I cried on the way home. My fellow students had no idea why she would have said this to me, and they comforted me as best as they could. At home I knew for sure that no, I did not want to be a yoga teacher. I finished my degree as a Doctor of **Naturopathy,** started building a client base for my Holistic Health practice, and gave

Reiki treatments (I had become a **Reiki** Master Teacher along the way). But even by doing all of that I was not making enough money; constantly I thought about other ways to bring in income to support my family and it was continuously a source of worry for me, yet at the same time I knew it would all fall into place eventually just the way it was supposed to. The only problem was that I am definitely not a patient person.

The divorce eventually got finalized, the kids had grown, K. moved out and rented together with his girlfriend. I wanted to sell the cabin and start over in a new place. I put the house up for sale and went looking for another property with my realtor. We had a lot of fun house-hunting, but there was no offer on my house yet. The real estate market had just started its long downward spiral. Over time we developed a friendship, and I told her my story and struggle to make enough money. She suggested becoming a realtor. I was a bit reluctant at first, but I realized that I could stay up here in the mountains working mostly from home and wasn't that what I wanted?

So off I went to Real Estate school. It took me just a few months to graduate and I hung my license at a local office, only ten minutes from my home. My house had received an offer and I found the "perfect" home, which all happened very quickly and in a miraculous way once again. After having searched for so long, when I opened the door to MY house I knew that it was the one. I had visualized it for a long time and it was exactly the way I had seen it in my dreams: cedar siding, log accents, brand new, loft, cathedral ceilings, open kitchen/living room, large unfinished basement for future projects.

The best part was the spectacular view of snowcapped mountains from almost every room; the way I would place my bed would give me the sight of the rosy glow of dawn reflecting from the high peaks. I got the house at a bargain price and moved in August 2005.

At the same time, my daughter decided to move in with her boyfriend. At first it was supposed to be just a trial during the summer break and before going to college. I was not happy but what were the choices? I could refuse and lose her altogether or I could let her go and we would still be best friends as we had always been. It broke my heart but I let her go. Here I was in the new home, 2300 square feet and all by myself.

"To stay present in everyday life, it helps to be deeply rooted within yourself; otherwise, the mind, which has incredible momentum, will drag you along like a wild river.-Eckhart Tolle

I immersed myself in work to avoid the burning feeling of loneliness. My entire life had evolved around my family and now, here I was alone with nobody to care for. Work and study became substitutes for closeness, and again, looking back I made the best use of a situation and walked forward on my path, going with the flow, accepting what I could not change and trying to see the positive in the situation.

PART 3

The best relationship is one in which your love for each other exceeds your need for each other.

~ *Dalai Lama*

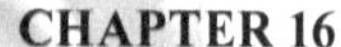

CHAPTER 16

It's All Coming Together

It all came together. My real estate career started off pretty well; the market was still producing some decent income. One day I got a call from our local Community College. Their yoga instructor had just quit, a few days before the semester started, and they asked if I could pitch in. "No way," was my answer. They begged and pleaded until I gave in but only committing to one semester until they found someone else. I had no idea what made me say yes and I was nervous; what I had gotten myself into? Never in my life had I written a syllabus nor talked in front of a group of people, let alone teach.

The first day of class arrived. My mouth was dry and I remembered the destructive words of my yoga teacher that I would never be a good yoga teacher because I hadn't been teaching from the heart. There were eight young women looking at me. Now what? To my surprise, I flowed through the class. I was open and honest with them, telling the truth that I had never taught before, but that I had 25 years of yoga practice to draw from besides of being a certified yoga instructor. At the end of our two hours together I was surprised how easy it all was. The girls were eager to learn, they had heard so much about yoga, good and bad, and they all were astonished that yoga was so much more than what they had perceived before. I was looking forward to the next class already.

"Yoga is an unspoken language. It comes from the silence and can be heard only by the heart." (Author unknown)

Six years later, the interest in yoga had grown tremendously. From one class with five or six students I now taught seven to eight classes per semester, and each class filled up just a few days after the schedule came out.

Some students came because they needed another credit, some came because they were curious, some because their doctors or physical therapists suggested yoga. Whatever their reasoning, all were welcome and sometimes, those who came "just for another credit" ended up falling in love with yoga and all its benefits. Some even wanted to become yoga instructors themselves.

In all those years I had never seen anyone who was not changed through their yoga practice. Most of these young people are amazed that yoga really is so much more than just the "weird" poses such as putting your foot behind your ear; that it helps them with stress relief, to calm their anxiety, deal with eating disorders, panic attacks before exams, and improve their posture and, more importantly, their outlook on life. Some of them even get so excited that they get their parents, friends, and family to try yoga.

The highlight of our classes was the fieldtrip to **Shoshoni yoga retreat**. For the beginner's yoga we went on a one-day retreat that consisted of **pranayama** (breathing) exercises, yoga postures, a delicious vegetarian lunch, and a tour of their beautiful land and temples. This again is a transformational experience for most students; they had no idea how peaceful people can live together, sustaining each other and the land, living simply, working, playing side-by-side and opening up their environment to the general public to get a glimpse that there is more to life than the daily grind.

It was a delight each time I read my students final papers with their comments on the retreat at Shoshoni, and it was encouraging for me that I was right on target with my life path—to give people choices, choices that can completely change their lives from stress to peacefulness, from fear of the future to hope and living in the present moment, from physical issues to health and vitality. Yoga is the answer to so many questions.

Then, for the first time in my career as a yoga instructor, my proposal for an Advanced Yoga class was approved and I took my first group of students through a weekend intensive Yoga Two class that ended, again, with the highlight of a Shoshoni fieldtrip. This time I had them experience an overnight stay with all that the retreat has to offer: silent meditation walks through deep quiet forests, a meditative hike up Rollins Peak, a soothing **Tibetan singing bowl** meditation, of course different yoga classes, chanting, pranayama and four delicious vegetarian meals in the cozy dining room overlooking the small pond, sitting next to the blazing woodstove. The world just stands still in a place like this. No cell phones, no computers, no worries. Just the here and now.

We did **Seva** (selfless service) in the morning as an exchange for the inexpensive rate that Shoshoni offers to college students. Some of us swept the floors, others washed dishes, polished the dining tables with natural citrus oils, or emptied the dishwasher; all the while the Shoshoni residents chanted doing their work.

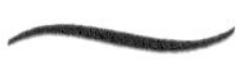

Happiness Is What You Are—Happiness is not a destination, it's a journey. Happiness is not tomorrow, it is now. Happiness is not a dependency, it is a decision. Happiness is what and who you are, not what you have. SSP

CHAPTER 17

All of these stories I tell you—about the teachings I've learned, the teaching I've done, and the places I've seen—are what prompted me to write for others to read.

So here I am in my bathrobe, a towel wrapped around my wet hair, straight out of the hot tub—yes, the hot tub. It is also where my best ideas and inspiration to write are coming from.

Sometimes writing can be a struggle, and it took awhile to decide what to include in this book. But one thing is for sure: it wouldn't be complete without the following two stories.

Love, Loss, Awakening

And you might guess, it's about men. To be correct, it's still a bit intimidating for me to write about this, which is why it took some time to develop the courage. However, both of these relationships are crucial to my development and who I am today.

I met the man who probably had the greatest influence on my establishment here in the U.S. during school. I was fascinated by the classes he taught about the great outdoors. At the time I studied Park Ranger Technology and everything that had to do with being in nature. I needed and craved this knowledge. From wilderness survival to water sports to maps and compass classes; I soaked the information up like a sponge. He was a great instructor who was passionate about what he chose to do and I thoroughly enjoyed his classes, his knowledge and expertise. On fieldtrips he made me feel safe and comfortable, especially since most of these classes had only guys enrolled and I was the only woman (and older for that matter, too).

However, when the separation from my husband happened I had to think of a better way to secure a job for the future, so with a heavy heart I gave up my Park Ranger studies and enrolled into a Graphic Arts Degree program. My former instructor and I had become friends in the meantime, and although I was not his student anymore, we kept going on outdoors excursions together, even including my daughter. He taught us how to cross country ski, canoe and many other interesting things that were necessary for us to spend time in the wilderness and be safe. It was a fun time and a tremendous relief from going through the stress of the separation and the drama of the ongoing divorce process.

I graduated with my Graphic Arts Degree and went onto the Holistic Health path, also at the same college. Our friendship deepened and we kept spending time together exploring Colorado's great outdoors.

After I graduated from the Holistic Health program I moved on to a four-year college in Denver. It was sad to leave my little college and its friendly campus, but in order to advance in my studies this was the necessary step.

My ex-instructor and I stayed in contact nevertheless. He had become my and my daughter's best male friend. But then something changed and I could sense a different kind of relationship budding between us. I had never thought about him in any other way than a friend, but suddenly something in the way we interacted with each other was more than a friendship. And then one day he confessed that he had been in love with me for a long time. He said that as my instructor of course he could not act on his feelings towards me, but now since I was not his student anymore he felt it was time to acknowledge and share his emotional state with me. It was and wasn't a surprise to me. I was still dealing with the fact that I felt discarded by my husband, unlovable, deemed to be alone, and then someone who had been my best friend for all those years told me that he is in love with me. It was just something that I couldn't comprehend right away. Yet it was a lovely moment and some of the scars that were still lingering in my heart started to heal. Yes, I had noticed that he was becoming friendlier towards me but I had not expected this to turn into a romantic relationship.

The entire scenario seemed to be perfect. We had been friends for so long, we had the same interests, and we were in love. My divorce was finalized a month after his confession of love towards me, and we decided to get married. Off we went on a wilderness canoe trip in the Boundary Waters, a longtime dream that both of us had shared. We got married on a small boat in what we called the "Wedding Cove," a sheltered cove surrounded by high trees with large boulders jutting out into the water that we had fallen in love with a few days earlier while exploring. It was a beautiful morning in July, and the sun was gracing us with her presence on our special day along with a light breeze. During the ceremony a pair of eagles glided in widening circles above us. It truly was a magical moment and, of course, the highlight of our trip.

The next day we took off on our honeymoon trip into the deep wilderness of the Boundary Waters where no motorized travel is allowed. It was a dreamlike experience. The profound silence brought me in touch with my very soul; I meditated with each paddle stroke in our tandem canoe. The only sound was the gentle splashing of water, the drops dripping off the paddle blade, an occasional faint call of the loon or the song of some other bird. No sign of civilization, just enveloped by pure, ancient, primordial nature. The stillness appeared sacred and I felt closer to the earth and my own deep inner self than I ever had.

We found a tiny little island that we chose to pitch our tent on for the night. Again, the silence was so profound that it made us whisper as to not disturb this extraordinary experience and to honor this special gift that we were receiving. A spectacular sunset was our entertainment for the evening, a dip in the cool waters of the lake before turning in for the night, and then we were lulled to sleep by the sound of gentle waves lapping onto shore. Suddenly the rainstorm came in. Without much warning, gale force winds were ripping on our tent and both of us had to hold onto the poles to keep it on the ground. The entire affair lasted about an hour. Mopping up the tent floor and reorganizing our belongings took another half hour until we finally got back to sleep. Another side of Mother Nature is what we had just experienced, all a part of the whole, yet a little different when there is no way out except by boat.

We had just gotten back to sleep when a loud splashing noise woke us up again, then some growling. A bear?? On our tiny island? It seemed he was trying to upturn our boat; although all our food was stored away in bear proof containers and hung high up in the trees, he might have caught some residue smell of something yummy and was exploring its origin. He was not interested in us at all, just tossed and played with our boat, which was our only way to get out of the wilderness, so yes, it was a little scary. What if he destroyed the boat? Or punched some holes into it? The entire event took about twenty minutes, but we knew there was not much we could do about it other than pray, and besides, it was a pitch dark night so we just sat in the tent, listening and determining if he was leaving or coming towards us. After a while we heard some more splashing and it seemed the bear had lost interest and left. Finally, we went back to sleep.

We woke up early to another beautiful rose and lavender-colored sunrise. But our main focus was to check on the canoe. Thank goodness it was ok, although there were some scratches and he did turn it over, but it still was secured to the tree that we had tied it too and no holes or other devastating damage had been done.

After a delicious breakfast (they always taste better in the wilderness anyways) of cinnamon oatmeal with walnuts and fresh brewed coffee we packed up everything to be back on the water before it got too hot or the afternoon rain set in.

My morning meditation took place in the canoe again, breathing in, paddle stroke, breathing out, paddle stroke. The lake was calm as a mirror; the only disturbance being the ripples that our canoe left behind. We glided silently through the deep, dark water, listening to the eerie call of the loons in the distance.

Our vacation continued that way for another week. The beauty of this ancient place was overwhelming and it was hard for us to even think about returning back home, but the day came to start the long four-day journey back to Colorado.

When we got home things had to be figured out about our future together. Up until that time we both had not really lived together, except spending long weekends camping, traveling or being at my house. And we both had lived alone for a very long time.

"The Inner Critic makes each of us a child. As we become the child in our relationships, we lose our sense of self. We are no longer self-contained, self-respecting adults. We look to others for validation. Our self-worth is based upon their opinion of us. Thus, everyone around us becomes a mother or a father whose support and approval is desperately needed to protect us from the constant criticism of the Inner Critic." Hal and Sidra Stone

It seemed that our wedding had changed the dynamics between us. From the friend and once student I had become his wife, yet there was still this teacher/student relationship lingering. Him acting "superior" and "teaching" me something all the time. It got to the point of becoming annoying. It was not an "equal" relationship.

I did what I usually do—I tried to talk it out, and when that did not work, I withdrew. Then things just got worse from there. I could not take off more time as I was working, but my husband had all those long breaks where he could do as he chose. He went on trips alone only to come home and "teach" me some more.

Long story short, we separated with the hope that giving each other space would solve the problem.

What happened? From being best friends, having the same goals, interests and dreams about the future to getting married to going back to friendship?

I had learned by that time that sometimes we just have to let all things work themselves out. Pushing solutions never really works. But other things happened and I could see how this was not what I really wanted; nor was it a good situation for either one of us. And then the feelings bubbled up again about being unlovable, discarded, something being wrong with me—another failed relationship—just what I needed.

We were friendly with each other, but basically went our own ways. Instead of growing together we grew apart. I focused on work as usual, since that had always proven to be my best therapy.

While my husband was on another long solitary vacation and not wanting to communicate nor compromise on our living situation, I moved into my new house.

Years went by and I got used to living alone again. We still communicated and occasionally spent time with each other, but it was not as it had been before. Over time we saw less and less of one another and I realized that indeed another relationship had failed.

Yet, I was happy by myself. I had lots and lots of friends and many interests besides of loving my job. And then, as it had happened to me many times before, when I feel content and my life is predictable and "in order," something happens.

Along came—THE ONE, the one who made me feel like a queen, who made me feel that I was all who mattered in the world and in his life—until he dropped me like a hot potato.

The entire "affair" went on over six rocky years with being apart more than being together. I was determined to make this relationship work and I tried EVERYTHING, and I mean everything, from giving him space to making a scene, from being patient to being pushy, almost to the point of changing my personality.

Here was the "teacher" again, in a different disguise—the greatest challenge that comes to us usually has to teach us something. This relationship definitely taught me patience and compassion, but also how to maintain self-respect in the end and how to forgive without giving myself up. Walking on egg shells and going from hot and steamy to cold and distant is not a good way to live; it is draining and self-destructive. Once again, if it wasn't for my daily yoga practice on all levels this relationship would have destroyed me. In the end the thing left to do was to walk away from it. It was hard, as there were so many wonderful memories too from when things were good and the hope that I had maintained over all those years that with my patience and love we could make this work. I realize now that nothing was my fault or even had anything to do with me; I could not "fix" anything.

I came to the point in my life where all the painful episodes of the past surfaced again and I had to ask myself some serious questions: were all the rejections, disrespect, ignorance and the scars they left on my heart and soul really necessary? Is this kind of suffering part of life? What purpose does it serve? I had to figure all this out, otherwise I would keep repeating the same patterns over and over again as I had done in the past. It was a hurtful process, but stepping aside and looking at it from an outside perspective gave a different view and understanding of what had happened.

There were uncomfortable questions I had to ask myself, but they were also crucially necessary. Once again journaling, mindful meditations, and calming, reassuring and familiar yoga practice helped me tremendously in the process.

I realized that there was still a lot of "residue" from my early childhood experiences left unaddressed. The rejection and lack of love during those important initial years kept me starving for love and acceptance. During deep meditation I got a glimpse of how to work through these issues. The questions that came up were: Do I really love and respect myself? Do I appreciate and honor myself? Do I allow myself to trust that there is someone out there who might love me? How about allowing myself more sweetness in life? Am I an overachiever? I mostly do things that have a purpose, and I rarely do things such as "just hang out," like so many people do. Why is that? Do I not deserve a break? Can I simply just do nothing but laugh and have fun? How can I expect others to love me if I don't really love myself? The final epiphany came again in deep meditation: I forgave those who couldn't love me nor accept my love for them, not because it was my fault, but because it's their own issues, and their own hurt and pain that are responsible for their actions and reactions.

Does that mean I have it all figured out? Does it mean that overnight all my problems disappeared miraculously? Absolutely not! It is a work in progress, and my story still unfolds, and there are days when all those emotional injuries bubble to the surface again and doubts creep up out of nowhere. But I have learned to accept them, not to dwell on them and remember the old adage "this too shall pass." Deep slow breathing, sending love, forgiveness and healing to myself with each in-breath and sending love, forgiveness and healing to everyone who ever hurt me because of their own hurt with each exhalation is a wonderful way to bring myself back into balance.

And the Story continues — Dealing with Death

How do we deal with death? Some of us believe in life after death, some don't. I had a sad conversation with a dear friend yesterday. He told me that he is severely ill and per his doctors, he has a maximum of two years to live. The illness is very aggressive and, there is no known cure currently available. My friend told me that he is at peace and that he accepts what is happening, and lives his life day-by-day. What matters to him, he said, is that he has something to look forward to tomorrow and that is all. Starting over every day. He was happy that we were spending time together sitting on his deck sipping wine, having a simple wholesome dinner and a loving conversation, watching the creek below, a pair of coyotes resting in the meadow. He is looking forward to tomorrow to see his dogs being happy and taken care of. But he also spoke about not believing in an afterlife. Our opinions differed on that subject. I have faith that nothing is permanent, not even death—and that we will be reborn. This provides me with peace. I spoke to him about a dream I had recently where we both were pure energy, pure consciousness, dancing together in the universe. Our energies that were pure love intermingling. There was neither male nor female, no time or matter. I told him that I would meet him there. It was a comfort to me, as it's hard to be faced with the reality of the death of a loved one. How do we start over with that person gone? But more importantly, how do we proceed and/or start over with this relationship right now?

What I realized through this conversation with my friend was that I did not know what to say, and that in turn made me really listen. It seemed that was what he most needed. Of course, it is difficult to talk and hear about the looming death of someone close but we need to give that person the space to express themselves fully without interrupting, without putting our emotions on display right there. There will be another time right for that, but I sensed all he needed was someone who would be totally present for him, who would just empathetically hold space for him. What is important, what isn't - enjoying the present moment, being mindful about every little detail, using time wisely.

I lost another dear friend several years ago where I was not as fortunate to spending more time with her. There were always other things to do: work, commitments, the distance on my part. On her part, doctor's visits, hospital stays, visits with her family. We kept putting off the days we had planned on spending together, thinking there was much more time. But there was not; she died quickly, sooner than anticipated. I remember being on a hike very early in the morning and suddenly could feel her presence around me. It was as eerie as it was special, and I knew right at that moment she had passed. When I got home I had an email from a nurse friend of ours that Jean indeed had died that same morning. Starting over meant missing my hiking/snow-shoeing buddy, my friend who I went rafting with and enjoyed strolling through art galleries and wine fests. She and I had met in school going through the Holistic Health Certification together. We spent many very close moments sharing our experiences. I miss her still, although it's been three years now.

A beautiful story from Hindu Philosophy

Parvati Longs to Marry Shiva

One day, when Parvati was only eight years old, her father, Himavan, took her to see Lord Shiva. From birth, Parvati had always been very spiritual. She always wanted to know about God, so she was thrilled to see Lord Shiva. But Lord Shiva was in a meditative consciousness and he did not pay any attention to the little girl.

After that first encounter, Parvati used to come every day to see Lord Shiva. She would offer him fresh flowers, hoping that one day he would open his eyes and speak to her. In the back of her mind, she had formed the idea that this was the man she wanted to marry.

The days became years and Parvati grew into a beautiful young woman. Still Shiva remained absorbed in his eternal trance. How could anybody disturb Shiva's trance? Once he enters into trance, he enjoys the highest and deepest bliss. So why should he come back?

One day, Parvati confided to her father, "I really want to marry Lord Shiva. He is meditating and meditating. How I wish that I could also meditate like him!"

Himavan was very sad that Shiva was not paying any attention to his beautiful daughter, who was so spiritual in every way. He decided to play a trick on Shiva: he invoked the God of Love to disturb Shiva's meditation. The name of this particular god was Madana. Madana had a bow and some arrows that were made of flowers. He used to shoot these arrows at his victims and then they would be filled with feelings of emotional love.

At Himavan's request, Madana aimed his arrows at Lord Shiva and the arrows fell as flowers at Shiva's feet. Suddenly, Shiva opened his third eye and caught sight of the god of love standing with his bow in his hands. Shiva immediately burned this unfortunate god to ashes because he had disturbed Shiva's meditation.

Meanwhile, Parvati was standing nearby with a most beautiful garland in her hands, but Lord Shiva did not pay any attention to her. It was as if she did not even exist. He simply closed his eyes again and went into trance.

Parvati's parents had witnessed the whole scene and they were furious with Lord Shiva. They felt that he had insulted their dearest daughter. "You cannot marry him, Parvati," they said. "This Shiva has been insulting you for so many years now. You must not waste your time on him any longer."

But Parvati would not budge. "I am going to stay here," she declared. "From now on, I shall eat only leaves, wet leaves." With heavy hearts, Parvati's parents returned home without their daughter.

For several years, Parvati stayed near Shiva, eating only wet leaves. Then she started eating only dry leaves. After a few more years, she gave up eating leaves altogether. When she gave up eating leaves, her name became Aparna, which means "one who does not eat even a leaf." Parvati became the goddess Aparna at that time because of her extreme tapasya, or spiritual discipline.

As time passed, Parvati went one step further. She stopped drinking water. She was living on nothing but air. Himavan saw that his daughter was becoming very weak. He knew that it was only a matter of time before she would die. So Himavan went to Lord Shiva and said, "Can you not see what you are doing to my daughter? All her life, she has wanted only one thing, and that is to marry you. But you have never even looked at her. If you are determined not to marry her, at least look at her. Otherwise, she will surely die."

Shiva condescended to look at Parvati, but to himself he said, "Let me test her one last time before I marry her." Poor Parvati had endured so many tests and still Shiva wanted to test her love and devotion. He took the form of an ordinary man and approached her. "You are such a beautiful girl," he said. "Why are you wasting your time here? I have heard that you want to marry Shiva, but what kind of man is he? He spends all his time in the cremation ground in the company of his ghost-friends. The garland around his neck is made of skulls. How can you marry someone as frightening as Shiva? Forget about him! Marry a normal man, like me."

Parvati's eyes burned. "What you are saying is untrue. Go away from here and leave me alone! I know who Shiva is. Do not throw your doubts and suspicions into me. I will never marry you, never! I will marry only my Lord Shiva. If you do not leave me alone this instant, I shall curse you!"

At that moment, Shiva assumed his true form once more. Parvati was so moved and overwhelmed to see him standing before her. Shiva said to her, "Any boon that you want, I shall give you."

"You do not know by this time what boon I want?" asked Parvati. "I want only to marry you."

"Granted," said Shiva.

After Shiva and Parvati were married, Parvati came to know that she had been Shiva's wife in her previous incarnation. Her name then was Sati and she immolated herself because her father, Daksha, insulted Shiva. But that is another story!

from The Earth-Illumination-Trumpets of Divinity's Home (Stories from the Indian Scriptures: the Puranas) www.Sri Chinmoy.org

by Sri Chinmoy

PART 4

If one advances confidently in the direction of his dreams, and endeavors to live the life which he has imagined, he will meet with success unexpected in common hours. He will put some things behind, will pass an invisible boundary; new universal and more liberal laws will begin to establish themselves around and within him; or the old laws be expanded and interpreted in his favor in a more liberal sense and he will live with the license of a higher order of beings. If one advances confidently in the direction of his dreams, and endeavors to live the life which he has imagined, he will meet with success unexpected in common hours.

~ ***Henry David Thoreau***

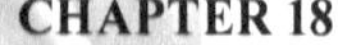

CHAPTER 18

Thoughts on Yoga and Living an Inspired Life Day by Day

In *Walking between Worlds* Gregg Braden states,

"Within the hearts of the children of forever lives the seed that each planted for themselves long ago. Their seed is a gift of truth, sleeping . . . . Awakened, that seed rekindles the ancient promise of those who have come before us: the promise that each soul survives the 'darkest' moments of life to return home again, intact and with grace. That promise is the seed of truth that we, today, have named Compassion."

And in the Dalai Lama's opinion, his only religion is compassion. Compassion is a word that we hear more and more lately, not only in religious terms or in the yogic tradition. What really is compassion? It is the opposite of anger. What is anger?

First, I think we have to analyze where the anger comes from. In many cases the source is the feeling of not being in control, which results in fear, which results in anger.

Once we can pinpoint the source we are better able to deal with it.

I find it important to be able to safely express that anger—vent, ask a good friend to just listen, and say the issues out loud. By doing this we can—most of the time—find the source of our anger and therefore solutions.

Personally, I rarely get angry. If you are like me, anger can take you by surprise. I learned that it is important not to beat yourself up over it. Anger is okay. We can't always be cheery, compassionate and happy.

Anger is our "shadow side" that is as important as our "happy side" and it will pass quicker if we just acknowledge it, safely express it, and deal with it, rather than suppress it. In Buddhism it is said that anger is one of the three poisons—the other two are greed and ignorance—and those are said to be the primary causes of the cycle of **samsara** and rebirth. Purifying ourselves of anger is essential to Buddhist practice. Even highly realized masters admit they sometimes get angry. For most of us, not getting angry is not a realistic goal.

Thich Nhat Hanh has a different view: *"When you express your anger you think that you are getting anger out of your system, but that's not true. When you express your anger, either verbally or with physical violence, you are feeding the seed of anger, and it becomes stronger in you."*

What Thich Nhat Hanh means here is that only understanding and compassion can neutralize anger. He suggests meditating/sitting with the heat of that anger. That too may not be possible for many of us.

And it was Buddha who said, *"Conquer anger by non-anger. Conquer evil by good. Conquer miserliness by liberality. Conquer a liar by truthfulness."* (Dhammapada, v. 233)

Now, back to the original question: What is compassion? Compassion is probably best explained by the Metta or Loving/ Kindness meditation, which is directing love and compassion first to ourselves with the following prayer:

"May I be happy. May I be well. May I be safe. May I be peaceful and at ease."

Then by bringing our awareness towards a friend or loved one:

"May you be happy. May you be well. May you be safe. May you be peaceful and at ease."

The next step is to direct the same prayer to someone we may know but don't consider a friend; next praying for someone out there in the world whom we don't know, just sending this prayer out to whoever might need it. The last and probably most difficult step for most of us is probably to send the same loving, compassionate prayer out to someone we might consider an enemy, someone who did us wrong, hurt or betrayed us. Those who are able to accomplish this last step have come a long way towards compassion. Compassion and patience go hand-in-hand, and are probably two of the hardest virtues to acquire, at least for me.

"Your worst enemies are your best teachers" is one of my favorite quotes from the Dalai Lama. There are so many opportunities to learn about patience, compassion and anger. My yoga teacher is one of those examples with her statement about me not teaching from my heart. I could have been angry; I could have given up yoga altogether; I could have yelled at her. Instead I took her words to heart, meditating on them but not letting them deter me from becoming who I am today. But maybe even more though, I developed compassion towards others. In situations where doubt, despair, fear or losing compassion creeps in, I chant **Om Namah**

Shivaya (I bow to Shiva). *Na* correlates to the earth element, *ma* to the water element, *shi* to the fire element, *va* to the air element and *ya* to the ether element; all five elements that our body is made of. By repeating and chanting the mantra Om Namah Shivaya, I am purifying my body, mind and spirit.

Yoga IS compassion: compassion to ourselves, and towards others.

"...Yoga enabled me to balance body, mind, and emotions, reminding me that through opening my heart I could touch the depth of my soul. Yoga became one of the greatest blessings of my life...... imagine consciousness in all its purity as a clear mountain lake. Gazing into the lake, we can see the mirror image of the mountains that surround it. This pristine illumination mirrors our Divine nature, and we experience love and oneness for all," said Nischala Joy Devi.

Feeling love, oneness and the interconnectedness of all of us, knowing that if I hurt someone else I am also hurting myself; being compassionate with each another—all this indicates that we are showing compassion to ourselves. Having the feeling to belong or giving someone that same feeling; that is compassion.

It is compassion that removes the heavy bar, opens the door to freedom, makes the narrow heart as wide as the world. Compassion takes away from the heart the inert weight, the paralyzing heaviness; it gives wings to those who cling to the lowlands of the self.—Nyanaponika Thera

Attachment

Attachment is probably one of the most common causes of unhappiness and suffering. We as human beings can get attached to so many things, some good, some not so good. We think that without the object of our attachment we will not be complete, happy or fulfilled. We can even become attached to our meditation practice; we expect a certain outcome, rather than allowing the freedom of the spaciousness of our mind to enter. Letting go, going with the flow, and the art of allowing are all antidotes to attachment. When we allow the power of pure consciousness to fill our hearts and minds with ease, there is not room for attachment, and we open ourselves up for divine things to happen.

"I looked in Temples, Churches, and Mosques. I found the Divine in my heart."—Rumi.

Everything is impermanent; nothing will last. Once we grasp this truth we can let go of attachment and free ourselves to live a life in mindfulness and emotional freedom. Everything we will ever need resides in our own heart and mind, such as the sanctuary we so long for, the safe haven, and the quiet place of bliss and peace lies. By letting go of attachment we free ourselves to re-discover that sacred place that has been inside of us forever.

"Nirvana teaches us that we already are what we want to become. We don't have to run after anything anymore. We only need to return and touch our own true nature. When we do, we have real peace and joy". (Thich Nhat Hanh, *The Heart of the Buddha's Teaching,* pg 140).

When we fully understand the nature of impermanence we will understand the value of the present moment, letting go of all attachments and free ourselves to experience true happiness. According to Thich Nhat Hanh, only through impermanence transformation is possible.

Belonging through Soul Connections

We all want to belong, and for many of us this happens through soul connections.

Have you ever met someone and instantly you feel a deep connection with them? You discover similarities in your lifestyles, likes/dislikes, the way you think and act and you KNOW that you know this person, although it's the first time you ever met?

Sometimes there is an "atmosphere" that feels charged, ripe with energy that you cannot explain. Sometimes it feels like you have known this person forever, or they may even feel like family.

It has been said that before we incarnate, we make agreements with certain souls for the purpose of exchanging energy, to learn from our experiences and sometimes come to peace with unresolved Karma from previous lives.

These encounters can be wonderful or not so wonderful; of course when they are pleasant we are happy and enjoy the experience, however, when we feel that we are dealing with unpleasant situations we will try to move away from them. It is to our benefit that we work through them, and the learning experience we find will bring us to the next level of our life path. There is something that we have to learn or teach to each other, and it is a valuable lesson for both people involved if we use the opportunity to grow.

We have "soul" families that we "agreed" to re-incarnate with, but there are also unfulfilling or empty attachments when we feel drawn to someone in an unhealthy way based on some kind of a contract in a past life that still ties us together; this is called a "negative contract."

The most important thing is to keep our compassion towards the other person, no matter if it is a negative or positive experience. There is a reason it is happening and we have our part in it.

Very few people have the privilege and honor to have a deep soul connection to another the way I described earlier; but those who do know exactly what a profound feeling of trust, love and belonging emerges from it.

Those very special friendships that we have need to be cherished, nourished and celebrated, even if we do not live close, see each other on a regular basis or even talk for years in some instances. I KNOW that some of these very sacred connections in my life will be there forever, and the moment we do reconnect we pick up exactly where we left off: days, weeks, months or in some cases many years ago—it is as if we just had spent time together yesterday. There is a deep knowing, understanding and yes, a "soul connection" that make this possible. I believe that some of us are connected on/at a different level of frequencies where time and space don't exist, where we realize that all that matters is the present moment that is to be lived, loved and utilized to its highest and best ability.

How are you?

"I am fine" is what most of us say. But are we really? Is it just a polite Question/Answer game?

For the most part it seems people don't really want an honest answer to that question. I noticed that when I first came to this country. Someone asked me how I was feeling and I started my answer only to be interrupted. So I realized quickly to just do the polite thing and give the answer that was expected. However, each time I do ask the question and someone answers "just fine" and I ask them "are you really?" more often than not people seem surprised and happy that someone really cares, and they will tell me how they feel. Most of the time things are NOT so fine.

On the other hand, I was also intrigued by the question and answer "I am fine," A lot of times when I do give that answer suddenly I DO feel fine, even though I may have been in a grumpy mood before.

I am not saying to be fake, but next time someone asks you how you are, think for a moment. And do the same when you ask someone how they are doing, and give them the gift of your presence, listening and care.

Some of my closer friends have picked up on my "concept" without me even really introducing it, but they KNOW that I care and that I really want to know what they are truly feeling and so oftentimes I get an "okay," "not so good," or a "medium" as an answer, and I know there is something they may want to share. My friends know that they can always tell me how they really feel and I feel honored by their trust. I feel equally blessed when they give me the same gift of letting me share my true feelings.

This is showing compassion too.

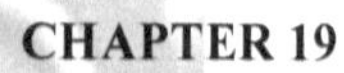

CHAPTER 19

Mindful at the Monastery

When I was invited to the celebration of Buddha's birthday by my wonderful Vietnamese student and her family, it turned out to be a long-awaited answer to my longing and praying. Deep in my heart I had this wish of belonging, being part of a **Sangha** (spiritual community). I thought I would never find it here. I thought I would have to go to India or some other exotic, faraway place—which I hesitated to do. After all, I made Colorado my home. My children and grandchildren live there and all my dear friends. It turns out that my Sangha was literally in my neighborhood, not even a half hour away and it had been there for a while.

It is said that when the student is ready the teacher will appear. I am ready now and the teacher (Thay Tinh Man) and the Sangha came into my life like a miracle. Once again it proved right that we attract what we project in terms of what we really want and need in our lives.

I was welcomed like an old friend, although I had never met any of these kind and gentle people except for my student. I arrived early, feeling a little lost as T. wasn't there yet and I knew nobody else. Slowly walking around the pond, taking in the spiritual, peaceful energy that was palpable everywhere, I was waiting for my friend when a lady walked up to me with big smile on her face and invited me to the English-speaking **Dharma** talk. Obviously there were not very many people there who were not Vietnamese, so I stood out a bit and she noticed me all by myself. How kind of her to approach me and invite me! I told her that I was to meet with T. at the koi pond, but we chatted and agreed to meet up later as she was also a volunteer at the monastery. I felt part of the community already.

After T. arrived we got ourselves some tea and settled into the meditation hall. I love the fact that in all spiritual retreat places it is common courtesy to leave your shoes outside; so there was a "wild" arrangement of all different kinds of shoes strewn all over the place in front of the door. I wondered if we would really all get "ours" back in this big mess. Some kind soul had built a cozy roaring fire in the huge fireplace that made the little building even more inviting with its crackling sound, warmth and light. We found our seats and then I saw K., my friend from earlier again. I felt so at home here already. Everybody smiled and made sure that I was comfortable. The room filled quickly and there was an atmosphere of calm excitement for the upcoming dharma talk.

Very quietly, the old monk walked into the hall, his hands in **Anjali mudra** (also called Namaste pose or Prayer position), which is widely used in the Asian tradition and accompanied by bowing towards each other. The gesture and the mantra "Namaste" mean "the Divine in me honors the Divine in you"—what a beautiful, peaceful greeting. Thay Phap An had the biggest smile on his face, and I think he smiled throughout the entire dharma talk. I remember thinking, *how can he do that? How can someone's constant facial expression be a smile?* I kept pondering the thought while the monk slowly made his way to his seat, and right there and then I decided to make it an intention to smile more often myself. Before Thay Phap An sat down he bowed to all of us again, just smiling, not saying anything. Everything seemed to slow down in this sacred environment and the presence of so many whose life dharma (purpose) is living mindfully, and extending kindness and compassion to everyone around them.

Very thoughtfully he took a sip of tea that someone had prepared for him, and then he looked around the room. I think he made eye contact with every single person present and his winning, loving smile made me feel very much at ease, welcomed and appreciated as it did—I am sure—for everybody else.

He greeted all of us and thanked us for coming and being part of the community. It was then I noticed his raspy voice and occasional cough. I wondered if he was ok and my thoughts started drifting off a little, thinking about a dear friend of mine who had passed away of lung cancer recently. But then he told us that he is from Houston, Texas and having problems with the current altitude. He had given many talks over the last few days at our monastery and in between he was on oxygen to recover. What dedication to his dharma and life path! How many of us would do that? I had deep admiration for this passionate old man already.

It turned out he was very funny, too. He told us that it took a little longer for him to get into the meditation hall as he had arrived and found all those shoes scattered around, and arranged all of them in neat rows. I know what many of us thought at that moment. But no, he did not want us to be ashamed—it was the beginning of his dharma talk about mindfulness. He invited us to slow down, to do every task consciously, even a seemingly unimportant one like leaving our shoes in a neat row. What does that say about how we live our lives, if we can't even organize our shoes?

After a woman hurried in late for the talk, making a lot of noise while finding her seat, chewing on a banana and dropping her journals, he went on to talking about doing one thing at a time and to stop multitasking, pointing out how we deprive ourselves of so many unique experiences because we do not pay attention to one single thing. It was not at all meant to be criticism, but a wakeup call for all of us to bring more awareness into our daily lives and to do one thing at a time. To do this one thing with full consciousness, even if it seems of little importance, i.e. putting our shoes next to each other or taking enough time to get to where we want to go so we are not late. How many of us watch TV while eating TV dinners, talking on the phone and reading at the same time. How often are our thoughts occupied with something completely different when outwardly we are communicating with someone? When was the last time you really listened to your partner in conversation rather than anticipating your answer or your turn to speak? How many irreplaceable moments do we miss in life just by not paying full attention to it?

The speaker system did not work properly. Someone in the back asked for the speakers to be turned up more. Thay Phap An smiled kindly and replied that they already were turned up all the way. Immediately two women took charge almost battling with each other to find the solution, one turned the device towards the back while the other suggested turning it to the side. Thay Phap An just smiled looking at the commotion and said just one word "RELAX." And then he said it again, calm and undisturbed, smiling all the way: "RELAX." So the speakers were turned half to the side, half to the back and all was good. Middleground?

We listened to his thoughts on relaxation, and about how slowing down whatever we do and discerning between what is really important and what is not can take a lot of stress out of our lives.

The chiming bell rang—the cue to close our eyes to meditate and simply breathe and be. Breathing in and breathing out, just keeping our concentration on the breath. *"The art of concentration is a continual letting go,"* Sharon Salzberg states in her beautifully written book *A Heart as Wide as the World. "We let go of a thought or a feeling, not because we are afraid of it or because we can't bear to acknowledge it as a part of our experience but because it is unnecessary."* It is as simple as that. Just focus on the breath. If a thought arises we let it go; it is not needed now. All that matters is this moment and our meditation—stilling the mind, turning in to ourselves. For the most part we think the same thoughts over and over again with nothing to worry about and nothing to lose. For now we concentrate simply on the emptiness of our minds.

Like A Star—At the end of the day, on the wings of your thoughts, go beyond the cares and troubles of the world. Remove your mind from everything and everyone, and become blissfully detached, like a star. Like a star, be free to radiate light, for your essence is light and peace. Enjoy the simplicity of the night sky, the peace. And then, when you want to, you can shoot down to earth. (Author Unknown)

I was filled with a tremendous amount of gratitude for being in the presence of this calm, kind, wise man, and even with my eyes closed I noticed that I was smiling. Smiling in meditation—that was new to me. My breath became deeper and slower throughout our time of deep silence, no thoughts, just the focus on breathing. As usual, when I meditate I lose the sense of time and the chiming bell rang again. We slowly opened our eyes to meet with the smile of our dharma master. The energy in the room was loving, quiet and very peaceful. We sat for a while before Thay Phap An spoke again, and in his slow, raspy voice he thanked all of us for coming together for Sangha and invited us to the actual celebration of Buddha's birthday. Some people got up right away, but he smiled again and reminded them to relax and slow down. I sat and enjoyed the presence of this man as long as I could. When I finally got up and walked outside with my new friends I looked in wonder at our shoes, neatly arranged in long orderly rows. I envisioned this frail old man who could hardly breathe on his knees doing this service for all of us. I hope it left an impression on everyone—just one mindful little thing, not only about arranging shoes in neat rows, but doing service to our fellow human beings in whatever small ways we can.

Meditation and Breakfast?

For me, meditation is one of the fundamentally necessary parts of my life. I cannot visualize my life without it and I start every day in meditation. Just as breakfast is the most important meal of the day, so is my morning meditation. No matter where I am or what busy day lies ahead, not meditating would be like not brushing my teeth or not taking a shower. Meditation is what keeps me centered, grounded, inspired.

I vary my practice according to my needs. Sometimes I just sit and follow my breath, other times I chant or silently repeat my mantra (a sacred, meaningful word) or gently gaze at an object that has special meaning to me, such as a beautiful rock, a pretty candle that a friend gave me or the first drawing of my children or grandchildren. In *The Yoga Sutras* Patanjali suggests to *"concentrate your mind wherever it finds satisfaction."* The key is to keep it simple and one-pointed; it should give you a sense of peace and enjoyment.

Mudras (hand positions used to focus in meditation) are another way to keep your mind occupied and focused.

Meditation styles will vary from person-to-person. What works beautifully for me might not work for you. Give yourself permission to experience. With time and practice everyone will find their unique meditation style. The important part is to be consistent. It will take time to establish your personal routine, but the goal is to make your whole life a meditation by taking one step at a time; starting with just a few minutes, extending to 10, 15, 20 minutes to an hour, and eventually giving yourself the gift of an entire day or weekend to immerse yourself in meditation practice. That does not mean you have to sit on your cushion all day long, but rather the opposite. Start by sitting and breathing right after you wake up, then mindfully making and eating your breakfast with your thoughts focused on what you are preparing.

Mindful Eating and Tea Meditation

Enjoy the smooth cool feeling of the apple you are about to consume, taste the crisp, fresh, slightly tart, juicy first bite becoming sweeter the longer you chew, and hold on to the lingering fruity aftertaste. Let your mind picture the apple tree in a large healthy orchard, visualize yourself picking the apple from that tree with gratitude in your heart. Make yourself a cup of tea and in your mind see the story that goes along with it, starting with the tea leaves thriving in a high cool Himalayan valley, and the gnarly hands, worn and tired from years of hard work, picking the leaves from the bushes, and carrying them in a basket to the village to be processed, packed and shipped to their destination. Visualize the fresh clean water you are about to boil and where it is coming from. Are you lucky enough to live in an area where you have your own well? Is it coming down from high alpine regions, charged with good energy? If not, you might want to bless the water before pouring it over your tea leaves to give it extra power. While your tea is steeping, allow your mind to become still and rest in thankfulness for all the abundance you have in your life. And finally it is time to enjoy your tea. Use your favorite cup, sit down on your cushion, hold the mug in your hands, feel the warmth, take in the fragrance of the steaming hot infusion, allow your gaze to follow the vapor swirling up into the sky, drawing beautiful patterns on the way, send a prayer into the universe along with it—then take your first sip. Ahhhh—tea meditation.

And so we go through our day, mindfully being aware of everything we do in every moment. Make up your own reminders to be mindful; for example, make it a habit to let the phone ring at least three times before answering it and let that be your prompt to use those three rings to take a few deep breaths. Make it a habit to get up a little earlier so you have extra time during the day. Take a moment when you wake up in the morning to smile—smile to yourself and the brand new day ahead of you. Position your bed so that you have a beautiful view as soon as you open your eyes. This is what sold me on my home. When I walked into the loft and looked out the window I knew that that was what I wanted to see every day first thing: a snow capped mountain range to the west that would glow in a range of rosy colors at every sunrise and tall, broad Ponderosa pine tree tops to the east, sometimes swaying gently in the morning breeze and being a home to countless birds waking me with their beautiful song day after day. At night, before drifting off to sleep, I can see the stars from my bed (and sometimes the moon shines so brightly that I feel like I am "bathed" in moonlight while sleeping).

I did not always have this privilege. I lived in apartments and in big cities with pollution, noise and crime, but I always made it a point to make my home into a sanctuary, no matter where I was—sometimes even a hotel room. It does not take much, just a plant that you like, a water fountain, a picture, an object from nature, or anything that inspires you.

Meditation for the Love of It

Sally Kempton in her book *Meditation for the Love of It* describes meditation techniques as portals into the underlying spaciousness of our minds that is clarity, love and innate goodness.

I truly believe that is exactly what we can achieve with our yoga/ meditation practice: clarity, love, goodness.

She reassures us that for meditation we don't need a special talent, but that the real key is in truly wanting to go deep. Kempton also speaks of our fear that we aren't "good" meditators. At one point, she writes that there is no such thing as "good" or "bad" meditation, but *"only our unfolding inner awareness and our relationship to the Self."*

Yoga and meditation are means for slowing down, for paying attention and for appreciation, which leads us into living more peaceful lives with ourselves and others and to open our hearts to the flow of grace.

What do we mean by grace? Kempton describes grace as *"the cosmic force that awakens the heart to its own vastness and love. Grace is the energy that connects to the ultimate truth, to the source of our being..."*

By opening ourselves up to grace it will express itself through the lightness and ease of flow in our poses, through the evenness of our breath and through the light in our eyes.

Once again, true yoga is not about aggressively forcing our bodies into twisted poses but to allow a natural change back to our roots of a simple meaningful life to take place. To just be and allow instead of do. When getting into deep meditation, *"The idea is to soften the stiffness that clings to your heart and to allow a feeling of inner surrender and tenderness to emerge,"* Sally Kempton suggests.

The Ragged Edge of Silence by John Francis has a beautiful passage that states, *"one must find a way to dismiss the ordinary, discursive mind, which is culturally conditioned."* He continues that this can be accomplished *"Through extended periods of silence, isolation, and fasting in the vision pit, a cave in the mountains or the desert."*

As much as I like this picture, the reality is that for most of us it is probably something that is out of reach in our modern world, but we can make small commitments of shorter periods of time where we withdraw from the media, phones, computers; we can fast for just one day (if no medical conditions would prevent us from doing so) or doing a juice fast. We can find a quiet place in nature to spend a few hours in silence and meditation, appreciating just what Mother Nature has to offer like the wind high in the trees, the soft murmur of a stream, the song of a bird. I have had my most profound meditations in nature. The outdoors simply is my favorite place to be. Without trying my thoughts dissolve into spaciousness, into the vastness of the sky, the depths of the forest and the flow of the brooks. Meditation comes naturally to me on high mountain tops or quiet valleys reflected in the slowing down of my breath, the deep love and reverence for life filling my heart as my body relaxes in the enjoyment of the moment. The richness of that experience is priceless and available to all of us. We just have to be open and receptive.

Sharon Salzberg in her wonderful and inspiring book *A Heart as Wide as the World* comments, *"While happiness is an end itself, one of the fruits of meditation, it is also the state of mind we can have right now, simply by respecting ourselves and living a life or caring. This is the happiness that is an essential ingredient for the ultimate liberation of our minds from suffering."*

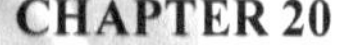

CHAPTER 20

Ease and Effort/ Sukkah and Sthira

"When we can accept all of life's contradictions, when we can comfortably flow between the banks of pleasure and pain, experiencing both while getting stuck in neither, then we are free."
Deepak Chopra

Think about those beautiful words from one of my favorite spiritual teachers, Deepak Chopra. What would life be if it were all joy and fun and happiness? How would we know if there were no days of doom and gloom? How could we define happiness if we had never experienced sorrow, pain and suffering? Yoga can teach us in many different ways to accept both, and not to get attached to either one.

Let's look at the physical poses, the **asanas**. There is always the sweet balance between ease and effort—sukkah and sthira, in **Sanskrit**. Our poses should flow with ease but we still want to engage our entire being, not just "hanging out" like rag dolls. However, we always honor the sutra of **Ahimsa** (non-violence) first and foremost, starting with ourselves by never going too far to the point of injuring ourselves, and of course extending the concept of non-violence towards others as well. However, we need to make the effort to perform our pose correctly and in alignment with full focus on the moment: what we are doing and why we are doing it. Most of my students are looking forward to **Savasana**, the deep relaxation, at the end of class. What a pleasure to let go, release, and melt and sink into your mat after all the physical effort of moving gracefully through your practice.

Vinyasa Yoga

Vinyasa yoga is one of the most joyful, dance-like, flowing styles of yoga. It is suited for all levels of yoga practice. For the total novice we flow very slowly yet gracefully, and as we get more and more flexible and gain strength along the way we increase the speed or hold the poses just a bit longer each time. Everything looks very easy and feather-light, but we ask the student if they feel like they really got a workout. Most will agree. Just recently I had another experience with a male student, a tall, strong, young man. After class he confided in me that he never thought that yoga would be "that hard"—what he meant was that it always looked very easy, not suited to develop strength and flexibility. Needless to say, he learned that his perception was proven wrong. I hear these stories again and again and each time I can't help but chuckle. Another example of ease and effort—yes, yoga looks graceful and easy but it does require effort.

Patanjali, the great Indian sage, lists nine obstacles on the way to yoga practice: illness, lethargy, doubt or impatience, resignation or fatigue, distraction, ignorance or arrogance, inability to take a new step, and loss of confidence. T.K.V. Desikachar in *The Heart of Yoga* explains that, "*these are manifested in symptoms such as feeling sorry for oneself, a negative attitude, physical problems, and breathing difficulties.*" Desikachar recommends **pranayama** (breathing exercises), such as a long quiet exhalation and a short pause after exhalation, as simple techniques to help overcoming those obstacles.

Take note of this excerpt from *Heart Yoga* by Andrew Harvey and Karuna Erickson: *"Watch your breath with steadiness and ease. The inhalation is absorbed evenly throughout the body, soaking in like moist earth receives a spring rain. Each inhalation flows right through you into the earth. Your exhalation smoothly floats out like dawn mist rises from a lake."*

Again, quieting the mind through conscious breathing and entering into deep meditation will help overcome obstacles as well, and we should not forget that yoga can take place in the mind. If we are ill and unable to do physical yoga, or sometimes not even being able to sit in meditation pose, isn't it still yoga if we spend our days contemplating healing thoughts, calming our minds and focusing on our breath?

CHAPTER 21

Inspired by GREEN

While I write this chapter, it is the end of May and finally I saw some budding trees this morning during my meditation walk. It looked like soft green lace had been laid over the landscape—suddenly there is green everywhere. It seems that all the plants just hovered underneath the cold surface of the soil and tried to stay warm and tucked away in their buds, braving the cold and wind that we had had just until now. Here at an elevation of 9,000 feet, weather changes so quickly from below freezing at night to the 80's during the day. Plants that survive up here are hardy and strong, yet flexible in their adaptation to the circumstances of the environment. Yes, even plants do yoga! Without flexibility they could not survive, without strength and the innate will to brave whatever comes along they would not make it up here. One of the topics the "mountain folks" up here talk about is that if the late frost doesn't kill it, the deer will eat it or the hailstorms during the summer will destroy what's left.

So yes, survival up here requires special skill: The will to try again. This is just as we try our pose again if we don't get the alignment right the first or second or tenth time; or when we start over during our meditation when we realize that our thoughts wander instead of keeping our mind still. It requires openness to new experiences, love for ourselves, our practice and others and the right attitude.

Green living is a large part of my life. I feel it is my responsibility to all life to live as green as I possibly can to save our planet for future generations. This deep love and respect for all of creation has developed since my early childhood, when I grew up in the perfect environment of my Grandmother's house and garden. I had the privilege to be raised on homegrown vegetables and fruit, to play in apple orchards and on green meadows filled with fragrant wildflowers. No pesticides were used in my Grandparent's gardens. Wherever I lived during the course of my life I undertook the greatest effort to start gardens and plant and harvest my own food. It was not always possible but even then I found ways to buy organic and local.

Probably one of the greatest challenges was growing food at the high elevation of 9,000 feet here in Colorado. I tried for many years, but until I put up greenhouses and cold frames it was a struggle and a battle that I lost for the most part. It still is a work in progress, as climate is very extreme up here from bitter cold to searing hot in a matter of hours, so I get a lot of exercise walking back and forth between computer and greenhouse, opening the doors and windows and then shutting them again according to the weather. However, it's a wonderful way of taking breaks from work and writing. Rather than trudging around an office building in a big city or along a busy highway, I am walking through the garden, pulling weeds, harvesting my veggies for lunch, watering, listening to the birds and observing the deer and big horn sheep wandering through the neighborhood—this is my walking meditation several times a day. Everything grows beautifully without any chemicals or harsh fertilizers—only horse manure and compost are used in my little paradise.

Of course, I only use natural cleaners. Anything that I have to buy to supplement my homegrown food is organic, and I am mostly vegetarian. I recycle, I live simply. I don't need lots of "stuff."

I buy most things that I absolutely need secondhand. Putting a sweater on rather than turning the heat up is a good way of saving money and the environment. My recent acquisition is a hybrid car. I traded in my gas guzzling SUV for a smaller, little bit older hybrid car, again helping to keep the air clean and money in my wallet. All of these things to me are just an extension of my yogic lifestyle. Some people think it is difficult to live the way I do. For me there is no other way and it is my way of living a healthy-inspired life. It makes me feel good to know that I do what I can to minimize my carbon footprint on this earth, and that I am doing the best I can to leave this world to enjoy for our children and grandchildren.

PART 5

"The basic thing is that everyone wants happiness, no one wants suffering. And happiness mainly comes from our own attitude, rather than from external factors. If your own mental attitude is correct, even if you remain in a hostile atmosphere, you feel happy."

~ ***H.H. the Dalai Lama***

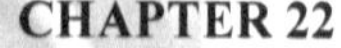

CHAPTER 22

Living an Inspired Life: What it Takes

Living in this manner definitely takes the right mind-set and attitude. We can choose, as there are always options. It makes a big difference if we wake up in the morning dreading to get up or the day ahead of us, or having an attitude of expecting a miraculous day full of wonders and love.

Looking at all the disasters that are happening around the world, it is a miracle in itself to wake up and to have options on how to proceed with our day. Isn't it just wonderful to be able to breathe? Aren't we lucky to have a bed to sleep in and knowing that we will have breakfast and running water for our shower? We take so many things in life for granted. That alone should be enough for inspiration, appreciation, and to be thankful for the little things in life.

The best way to make our day a good one is (of course) to start with some quiet contemplation, which we should allow to lead us into meditation. Meditation, as we have seen, is something very simple such as paying attention to our breath. Sometimes I feel like experimenting a little: for example, I found a beautiful old Tibetan singing bowl in a tiny little store close to my hometown that I had not noticed before. Driving by recently I decided to stop and check it out. What a gem I had discovered. There were four singing bowls for sale. I tried them all, but two particularly caught my attention with their beautifully striking, long vibrating sound. Needless to say, I bought one and brought it home. I played a little with it yesterday and combined it with the bowls I already had.

This morning I woke up early and just knew that my daily meditation practice would involve my new singing bowl. I took it outside and played it near the wind chimes. It was a blustery morning with the sound of nature represented in the summer wind and reflected by the gentle ringing of the chimes in the breeze. I slowly ran the striker around the rim of the singing bowl, increasing the vibration and sending prayers of peace and love out into the world. These harmonizing sounds automatically make us slow down, close our eyes and sink into our own sacred space—even if it is just for a few moments. It started my day peacefully and, literally, with a good vibration.

Like all forms of meditation, playing singing bowls requires that we stay fully present during the process, rather than focusing on any outcome. In doing so, we release any inhibitions or expectations of "what needs to happen" so that our thoughts can flow freely and creatively.

Most mornings start with my walking meditation. What is the difference between an ordinary walk and a walking meditation? The answer is "Awareness, consciousness, mindfulness, breathing." This particular morning the air was crisp and cool, despite being a summer morning in late June. Yet at 9,000-feet this is not unusual. Breathing in this wonderful cool, fresh, clean mountain air in itself is a blessing and makes me smile. Naturally, the breath slows down in order to savor and enjoy every bit of it. Slowing down the breath automatically slows down the mind and all its chatter as well, making space to focus on the beauty around you. The tall majestic mountain views, vibrant green leaves on

Aspen trees, the crystal blue Colorado sky, the cheery morning song of the multitude of birds. And then I noticed my friend, the little red fox, who accompanies me on many strolls throughout our neighborhood. Again, just watching him made me smile. First he patiently hunkered in front of a gopher hole, waiting for his breakfast to appear. When that did not seem to happen, he got up, wandered up the hill and started playing with pinecones before rolling in the dirt to start his morning cleaning ritual. Next, he ran down into the bushes just to continue licking and grooming himself before dozing off into his little fox nap and dreams. I stood in wonder and with gratitude for being graced with this experience. Naturally a mindfulness meditation came to me.

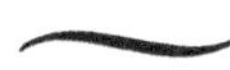

Breathing in the fresh crisp mountain air—Breathing out I am happy—Breathing in gazing upon the distant snowcapped mountains—Breathing out I feel gratitude—Breathing in I know we all are breathing the same air—Breathing out I know you are my friend. SSP

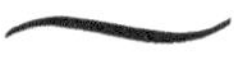

On other days we may prefer to really just be quiet and allow ourselves to sink into the stillness of our own heart; it may be for just a few minutes but sometimes sitting for an hour or longer seems appropriate.

Setting an intention in the morning just for this day is a good way of living mindfully and inspired. How about smiling more? How about dedicating one day to not complaining? How about trying to say something nice to everyone we encounter during the course of the day? When we meet with a friend or talk to them on the phone let's try just for once to listen, to really listen to what they are saying. This is a wonderful gift we can give to someone, and it will change the course of the conversation and the relationship. For the most part we are too concerned with ourselves and not with others. We "pretend" to listen, but do we really? Most of the time, we think about what WE want to say instead. How much more pleasurable it is to experience the joy and gratefulness in the eyes of our partner when they realize that they are being listened to, that they matter?

Or try adding one "green" action every day. For example, we could decide to buy one item organic that we would buy anyways. That is a start, as it not only helps the environment but is healthier for us as well. Or start recycling and choose to home cook meals instead of eating TV dinners out of convenience. Just spending a few hours of joyful cooking can be an inspiring experience on its own with the benefit of freezing some of it and VOILA, here are your pre-cooked, homemade healthy meals for a few weeks. Not only will we live healthier but we will also save money and have control over what we eat and what is in it. Again, it's the little things that make all the difference in our lives.

"Just become quiet, still, and solitary, and the world will offer itself to you to be unmasked; it has no choice. It will roll in ecstasy at your feet." Franz Kafka

Creative Visualization

Many years ago, another book had a great influence on me when it came to directing my life. *Creative Visualization* by Shakti Gawain. I read the book and started listening to the accompanying cassette tape (yes, it's that long ago) on a daily basis. The concept is still valid today, based on the idea that we attract what we think about, that we have total control over our thoughts and that we can choose to have some control over the direction that our lives will take. In fact, this tape was the start of my long inspirational journey to the place where I am now.

I am a big fan of the **Law of Attraction** in whatever way, shape or form. There are so many wonderful people out there teaching this life-changing art form. It is amazing how simple the concept is, and how it is available to all of us at any time. For me, the beauty that lies in it has to do with controlling our thoughts and taking charge of what we really want, and only focusing our awareness on those thoughts and ideas, avoiding any negativity. However, it is not a forceful technique; rather, it is based on allowing and appreciating. It is not a new concept by any means, but rather has been cradled within yoga philosophy for thousands of years by stilling the mind, avoiding violence, and concentrating on the good. Most great things in life that have value have been around for a long time and are mostly free. I find that fact rather refreshing. No, money is not the guarantee for happiness. It does help, but I know a lot of people who have a lot of it and are mostly unhappy, worried, even angry.

What matters most is how we live day-by-day. Do we feel good about our deeds? Were we of service? Did we make a difference in the life of another?

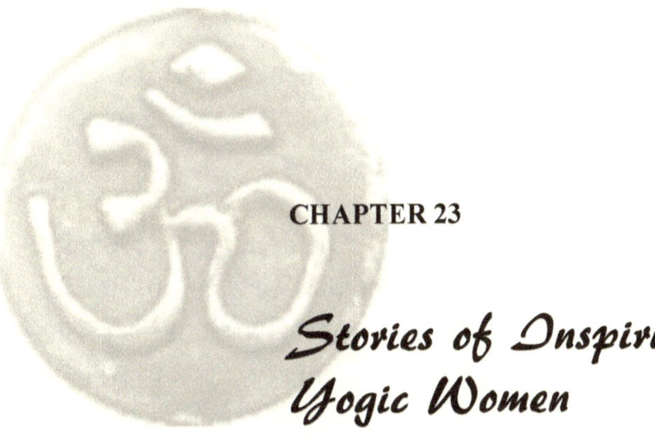

CHAPTER 23

Stories of Inspiring Yogic Women

Kathy Mastroianni, RScP

Life. Why are we here? Why are we put on planet Earth? To learn? To love? To Be? As I think through my life, I wonder . . . and I remember . . .

It was September 2, 1972. Summer vacation was nearing its end. I had just turned six-years-old, and just days before my mother hosted a very fun birthday party for me. Friends, relatives, cake, games. What a great day! School was about to start and I would be entering first grade. Still nervous and shy, often hiding behind my daddy's legs, I was also excited to see what the new school year would bring. The day was overcast, yet hot. Daddy was at work. Mommy was in her bedroom and my sister, Carol, who was 11, was already outside in the back yard. I ran down the stairs and yelled, "Mommy, I'm going out to play." I shut the door and the house grew silent. And then there was a shot.

A short while later, Carol came into the house and found our mother who had killed herself. Our lives would be forever changed and influenced by that moment, by that event. Much later I learned that my mother was in an abusive relationship with my father. She had turned to drinking to numb the pain and to escape. She tried to leave. In the early 70's there were no shelters. There was no one to help her and nowhere to go. She felt like there were no other options so chose the only way out she felt she had.

Later, when I was 14 and my sister 19, our father died of a heart attack. My sister became my legal guardian. The aunts and uncles would say, "You girls need to stick together." Through many ups and downs, we have stuck together and are very close, even with Carol in Michigan and me finding my way to the mountains of Colorado. Life has been a journey, for sure. A journey towards service, wholeness and love.

Fast-forward to 2011. I am Chief Executive Officer of a rural emergency women and children shelter. At 44-years-old, I am so blessed to fill-in the full circle of life. To provide brave women and children and even their pets who have the courage to leave abusive situations with a safe place to go. Looking back, my mother was definitely my inspiration for doing what I do—I dedicate my job to her. Now, my beautiful, amazing daughter who is 11-years-old is my inspiration. I need to be strong and model a healthy life for her. I, too, was in a very unhealthy marriage and after 17 years got a divorce. It was a long and painful process, yet I knew that the lessons I personally learned would be used to help others to be stronger and to grow.

I love what I do because I see the beauty and light in everyone who is in the midst of crisis. Even when they feel that there is no other answer. No solution. No way out. I so completely honor their courage that it takes to leave abusive relationships. To step from the known (abuse) into the unknown. Stepping through fear to freedom. It is so powerful! The other amazing part of doing the work that I do is watching folks blossom. Knowing I can make a positive difference by giving people encouragement in their times of seeming darkness. By helping them see the light and a little bit of the endless possibilities that are beyond. Years later I will talk to people and see the HUGE difference in their lives—and then watch them pay it forward to help others.

The greatest challenge to my job is that it is 24/7. I have had to sacrifice family time and sometimes just having the freedom to do things for me or my family or now my house. It is not Monday-Friday 9-5. A crisis can be anytime and as the CEO I need to be there for staff and volunteers, so even when I am "off"—so there is rarely any "off."

Looking back and looking forward, I would definitely do it all again. It has helped me to become who I am, and I like me! It has been a great personal growth experience and even with the seemingly most difficult situations, it is filled with hope. It is a work of heart. I also love that I can show through powerful actions to my daughter that we all can make a difference in our world and we are here to help each other.

My future is evolving in wonderful ways. I have found great joy in deepening my connection to Spirit—my God Source. Through the powerful practices of Yoga, meditation and the many wonderful teachings at my spiritual community, I look forward to my continued expansion as a Spiritual Counselor and supporting others on their spiritual journey—their journey inward to their true Self which is pure love, amazing joy, and of course, Peace. Together, we can create peace in our own lives and in the lives of others—and then it spreads to the world.

Kathy can be contacted at 303-838-2047 or at mastrokj@aol.com if you would like to learn more about her spiritual counseling practice.

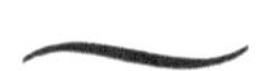

Mira Paul (Student of Environmental Studies, Red Rocks Community College, Lakewood, CO)

My moments of greatest inspiration come when I am climbing mountains. I'm not talking about the gently sloping trail through the woods and up to the crest of the hill; no, I'm talking about vast, rocky and treacherous mountains, where Mother Nature dictates your success or failure, where, to the untrained eye, no living thing exists. But if you look hard enough, these mountains are an ecosystem all their own: tiny flowers, grasses and greens cling stubbornly to the fleeting summer months, tiny spiders crawl amongst rocks on a 14,000-foot summit, and rodents whose cheeks are stuffed with grasses and lichens prepare for the ever-threatening winter. The scene on a high mountain peak is panoramic. Every direction you look are snow-flecked mountains, lush valleys and bubbly cumulous clouds scattered in a rich blue sky, and if you stretch your hand high enough, you sometimes can touch the base of a cloud...how many people can say that they have done that with their feet still on the ground?

Not only is the aesthetic value of these mountains my inspiration, but also the physical, mental and emotional challenge they pose. Oxygen is minimal at this altitude, wind and sun scour exposed skin, and temperatures fluctuate without warning. Altitude sickness is a constant threat, even to the acclimated and seasoned climber. It takes a great deal of mental toughness and yes, stubbornness, to reach the summit. You must learn to pace your breathing, your heartbeat and your steps all in unison; then you will find a rhythm, almost a drone, that pushes you to the summit. That's what climbing is all about: pushing yourself to your very limit and then beyond, to where you thought you would never be able to go. Only now you've been there, and you know you can do it, and next time, you can push yourself even further.

High-altitude mountains separate the strong from the weak. Not only must you be physically strong to climb a mountain, but also mentally and emotionally strong. When your muscles scream for you to stop, and your lungs cry for oxygen, and your heart threatens to leap from your chest, and your only relief is to quit, you must find that calm mental voice that forces your physical being onward. But along with this mental strength comes the discipline to know when a successful climb is not in the cards. You cannot get "summit fever" at the expense of your life; you must have the courage to turn around when the weather, for example, is looking bleak. Live today, climb tomorrow.

High-altitude climbing combines discipline with physical, mental and emotional strength. The personal well-being that infuses me when I climb is priceless. When I climb, I am in my happy place. It is almost like a meditation. Right foot forward, inhale, left foot forward, exhale, right foot forward, inhale, left foot forward, exhale. I love how my heart pounds against my ribs, how I create a perfect song, and my lungs, heart and boots are the instruments.

Desiree Rumbaugh, Certified Anusara Teacher

I knew Yoga was going to play a very important role in my life on the day I took my first yoga class. I felt something moving inside my heart and soon felt tears running down my face during the standing pose, Trikonasana. I did not understand it on a logical level of reason, but my soul knew I had come home. It was 1987 and I was 28-years-old. Having been a dance teacher for many years, it wasn't long until I was pursuing Yoga Teacher Training

Courses. Yoga was healing me, where dance was starting to break me. I knew I had to shift.

I am practicing and teaching yoga because I love it. I could say I am living a life of service, but I also realize that it is absolutely serving me as well. I have befriended my body and I am slowly healing old wounds. As I continue to practice, it feels like I am peeling back all the layers of myself, and getting closer and closer to my inner Being.

Now the greatest challenges for me are showing up, as my body is signaling that I need to take more time off to replenish. Even though I love what I do, it can still be done in excess.

When I began my traveling teaching career, I used to identify myself as a wife, a mother of two children and a yoga studio owner. Life taught me a lesson about identification because shortly thereafter, my husband and I divorced. In the 18 years we had been married, we had grown apart and become incompatible. My Yoga practice was asking me to be more honest and authentic, and clearly it was time for us to go our separate ways. Now my identity statement was reduced to mother of two children and yoga studio owner. I proudly announced that at the beginning of my workshops.

I was moving along, flowing with all the bumps and opportunities that occur when one embarks on a major life change at 41, and then, 3 years later, my eldest child, my only son, was murdered at the age of 20. This plunged me even deeper into my practice, looking for some kind of respite from the unbearable pain and also drew me closer to my younger daughter. Because she was about to go off to college, I threw myself even more completely into my traveling teaching career. Sharing my story with the greater Yoga community was definitely helpful. I learned, most of all, that I was not alone, which was oddly comforting.

As time went on, I drew some sense of solace from the feedback I got from others that my ability to stay strong (while also showing my pain) was inspiring to them. For three years after his passing, I was still wrestling with reality and I shared that struggle in my workshops. After three years of fighting it, I finally found a way to allow it to be. It is said that we become different every seven years. It has now been seven and one-half years since that time, and I do believe that I have changed in terms of my views on life and death and my ability to understand the deeper mysteries that are a direct result of this journey. I would not wish it on anybody, but I am happy to share my story with anyone who finds themself in this place.

I have learned to co-exist with the reality that my son's soul needed to move on earlier than I had ever expected, and I have been able to come to a place of peaceful acceptance rather than bitter resistance. I have been able to completely let go of needing to identify with being a mother of two children to be OK in the world. I am OK being a mother of one angel and one living child. That took a lot of work. I had to learn to meditate in order to connect with my identity as spirit more often than my identity as human. This is not to say that identifying with one's humanity is a bad thing. It is absolutely necessary while we live on earth. And . . . of course it comes with attachment and that is what causes suffering---strong attachment to temporary things and people.

A few years ago I gave up my yoga studio to be a full-time traveling teacher. Funny how my once proclaimed "identity" has shifted.

Recently I re-married, which was for me, definitely a spiritual milestone. It is blessed evidence that tremendous healing is happening, and it means I am learning to trust Life. There has been a significant change in how I introduce myself. I now just give my first name.

Ever since I was 35 I have had the dream of creating or belonging to some kind of community that would grow older together. My longing for community of like-minded souls is partially fulfilled as I travel the world and make new friends every week. The next phase includes learning how to create something more local and sustainable. After all those years of airplanes and living out of suitcases, I long to get my hands in the dirt and grow my own food. I love the idea of making the everyday life sacred and celebrating the aging process with good friends.

I have to agree with Joseph Campbell when he said, "follow your bliss." At the very least, you will enjoy each day of your life. Of course it takes courage to say no to temptations in order to live a more conventional life of conformity. But all those who are born with a longing for something different are encouraged wholeheartedly to boldly go and follow that road less traveled. I would tell people to trust Life as it unfolds, even if it hurts sometimes. Of course there will be pain, but one thing I know for sure, we are never abandoned. Grace is everywhere, supporting us through nature and other people. Trust Grace and Follow Your Bliss. Best advice I have to offer.

http://www.desireerumbaugh.com/Desiree_Rumbaugh/Intro.html

~

Carrie D'Angelo, Inspiration Through Challenge

Inspiration reveals itself to us in a number of ways and when we least expect it. It can greet as a gentle breeze, or as a powerful storm that washes away the very landscape we have grown accustomed to. It is not something that can be bought or forced, but when the time is right, it hits you and there will be no denying it. It's an absolute gift of divine proportions.

It took me many years, and what felt like a lifetime of deeply challenging experiences to finally begin to embrace my gifts, a passion found by an unexpected source of inspiration. It came to me at a point in time when I felt I couldn't handle one more thing. I didn't understand why life had to be so difficult and why every direction I chose to pursue seemed to lead me down another path of hardship and emotional turmoil. I would have never fathomed that all these seemingly difficult events would lead to that very moment when it would all began to click.

It came as a call in the early morning hours: "Carrie, you need to come home." It was in that very instant my heart sunk through the floor. My eyes began to well up with tears as deep sobs came pouring out of my soul. I gripped the steering wheel tightly as I drove past the barricaded intersection that I had stopped at earlier, only to be turned away with no answers.

The tape was still strung around the accident scene while the last of the cleanup crew was busy trying to reopen the road. I tried to focus, but was barely able to see beyond the tears filling my eyes. I found myself in a surreal haze questioning everything. *This can't be happening to me*, I kept telling myself, *maybe he just ran out of gas? Maybe he was broken down by the side of the road somewhere? Maybe his cell phone just died?* I was in a state of shock and denial manifesting in a whirlwind of emotions.

The knots in my stomach intensified as I approached my house. I pulled in the driveway as his parents sat on the front porch awaiting my arrival, their faces struggling to maintain composure. They embraced me with a warm hug and suggested we go inside. The fear began to grow in me as I placed my hand on the handle. Slowly opening the door I prayed that I'd see him standing there but all that greeted me was a lifeless house filled with stacks of unpacked boxes. I fell to my knees as the most gut-wrenching sadness raced through my very being. Just then it hit me, this was really happening…he wasn't coming home. It was my love and partner that was in that tragic car accident and it was there he breathed his last breath.

Many months passed before I began to accept that he was gone from this reality. But was he really? I couldn't see him, but I could feel his presence everywhere. In a sense it was as though he had never left, as though he was watching out for me. Every corner I turned there was some sort of "sign." I began seeing 11:11 constantly on digital clocks and 11's on license plates, addresses, mile markers—there was no escaping it. I knew it wasn't just mere coincidence. I began immersing myself into anything I felt could provide me answers, an understanding of what I was seeing and experiencing. Countless days and hours I spent researching, reading, and learning to find stillness and peace within myself. The more time I devoted to this, the more I began to see clearly. My senses were awakening. I could feel myself changing from the inside out. I began to see, feel, and know people at a level I never knew possible. It was as if a barrier had been lifted, a veil to a once hidden world.

It was during this time that my gifts of channeling spontaneously awoke. Words began flooding my mind as I received pages upon pages of wisdom about life and my purpose. People began mysteriously appearing in my life, seeking my guidance during their times of crisis. It became a deep passion of mine to help and provide others with insight that may awaken their divinity within as well. It was as though a gift was bestowed upon me to be of service to others. It became a spark that ignited my soul until it enveloped the very essence of who I am. It filled me with energy and a sense of undeniable joy.

This ultimately lead me to creating Token Rock, an inspirational organization and Web site comprised of all the information I had gathered during those months of soul searching . . . . a place to find comfort and understand why we experience the things we do. How to see the beauty in the most difficult aspects of our lives, knowing that there is purpose and a destined path; that we're not here wandering aimlessly without a guiding hand.

Today I continue to grow and expand my own knowledge and awareness through tokenrock.com, as well as providing intuitive counsel. As co-founder of this growing organization I have been blessed to collaborate with insightful contributors from all over the world, many of which are experts in their field of study. Together we are on a mission to provide knowledge and inspiration to humanity. All of this sprouted from the seed of a seemingly tragic experience, only to blossom into a magnificent life experience.

This was my partner's gift to me...he left me a trail of bread crumbs to follow, one he knew that would awaken me to *me*. In his death I found my inspiration. For this I am ever grateful.

Carrie-Anne D'Angelo

Self-Empowerment Coach, Intuitive Guide, Writer and

Co-founder of Token Rock—A webby nominated Self-Empowerment and Inspirational website http://www.tokenrock.com/ http://Carrie-AnneD'Angelo.com

Token Rock, 20165 N 67th Ave, 122A-187, Glendale, Arizona 85308 - 480.961.6811 | Office - 480.753.4574

deZengo Moore

My introduction to yoga began in Seattle, arriving at a crucial point in my life. Beginning just prior to a diagnosis of stage III/advanced breast cancer and in the midst of an extremely toxic and financially devastating four-year divorce, yoga made a huge impact on my own ability to survive and recover. During chemotherapy treatments, it took everything I had to walk the few feet needed to reach open space and connect with nature, while confronting my broken spirit and body. The impact of yoga in my life has been incredibly positive. Allowing me to once again feel full of compassion and with a desire to give back. Now, through the Internet, we can see so many using adversity to create positive change, such as Sophia shares in her book. It is wonderful to be a part of that change.

deZengo Moore, Health & Wellness Editor OM Times Magazine; Yoga & Zumba Instructor, Artists, Graphic Designer, Social Activist

Jenny Kachnic, CCMT, CRP, Author

From the time I can remember, I always loved being around dogs. I used to dream of becoming a veterinarian someday and spending all day with them. Like a lot of us, I ended up doing something very different with my life: accounting and office work.

I always made it a priority to keep animals and dogs in my life through my volunteer work. I have trained dogs, cared for them, helped them get adopted and promoted wonderful animal causes throughout my life.

After a couple of decades of reluctantly working at unfulfilling jobs, I decided it was time start living and to finally make my passion my way of life. Happiness is a choice, and I made the choice to devote my life to animals, specifically dogs. Once I took the first step, doors started to open for me that I never thought possible. That was my sign that I was finally living my true purpose.

I wanted to teach people about how to care for their senior dogs and inform them on all the options for them that I discovered through my journey. I now had the courage to finally write that book I always dreamed of.

Now I get to wake up excited about my day, as I know I am making a difference in the lives of dogs and the people who love them.

CANINE WELLNESS, LLC www.CanineWellnessSite.com 303-324-3911

Editor and Author of the forthcoming book—Your Dog's Golden Years—A Manual for Senior Dog Care—Including Alternative and Complementary Options.

PART 6

When you dance, your purpose is not to get to a certain place on the floor. It's to enjoy each step along the way."

~ ***Wayne Dyer***

CHAPTER 24

Food for Thought (from my daily inspirational emails)

Giving, Being, Receiving

Most of us want more in our lives, more appreciation, more attention, more love, more money, more happiness, more time…

The more we are willing to give, the more we will receive. But we have to begin by giving to ourselves. Give yourself more time, more attention; give yourself more love, and more of what you want from others, or from your life in general. Then decide how to offer this "more" that you have to the world, and you will receive even more back in return. In Reiki we learn that in order to pass the Diving Healing Energy on to others we ourselves must be filled up with it first, and then the "overflow" will go to others as well.

Awakening

—See and feel everything whether it's labeled good or bad with clear, intense awareness, an open heart, love and compassion. Notice more what you usually try to ignore. As you awaken more and more to the wealth of feeling and inner wisdom an unknown passion with feelings of love, sensuality, gratitude and joy will

fill your entire being. The intensity of the experience will be a blessing beyond expectations. SSP

"Undisturbed calmness of mind is attained by cultivating friendliness toward the happy, compassion for the unhappy, delight in the virtuous, and indifference toward the wicked." The Yoga Sutras of Patanjali

"The underlying purpose of all the different aspects of the practice of yoga is to reunite the individual self with the Absolute or pure consciousness—in fact, the word yoga means literally "joining." Union with this unchanging reality liberates the spirit from all sense of separation, freeing it from the illusion of time, space and causation. It is only our own ignorance, our inability to discriminate between the real and unreal, that prevents us from realizing our true nature." The Sivananda Companion to Yoga

Through the practice of yoga I have found many wonderful likeminded friends; "True Friends," as I call them. What do I mean by a True Friend? There are many levels of friendship and the word "friend" is sometimes used very lightly. I believe a true friend is very rare. True friendship means 100% trust in each other, knowing that they would do anything for each other, even if it would mean giving up one's life for each other. True friends can share EVERYTHING, good or bad; being a real friend means speaking the truth, even if it hurts. True friends will make time for each other when the other is in need of their company. They are likely to be interested in all aspects of each other's lives and will not desert each other for other people.

A true friend is someone who would stop their own life to help, despite the fact that there was no incentive or even risk or pain for them to do so. A true friend knows everything about you and still loves you, if not more so. That is true friendship to me and it ranks at the same level with true love, which is as powerful as true friendship, and the two combined create the ultimate in human relationships.

"When we open ourselves to the heart of a friend or lover, we trust that we are cherished, loved unconditionally."..."Let there be no purpose in friendship save the deepening of the spirit." Khalil Gibran

What do you REALLY want for Christmas?

The answer to this question will change over the years as we grow older. From all the material things that could not bring us REAL happiness, we may have finally arrived where we can clearly see what matters.

What do you really want for Christmas this year? If we are coming deep from our hearts, in thinking about giving this year, could we seek to give more grace, kindness and gentleness? Could we spread the joy that comes from being deeply rooted in a belief system/faith? How about opening our eyes and hearts to receive true beauty by being mindful in every moment, appreciating all the little things that we so often overlook? How about cultivating an attitude of gratitude?

~

Christmas is not as much about opening our presents as it is about being quiet and listening, opening our hearts to allow love to enter. SSP

~

May the spirit of Christmas bring you peace, the gladness of Christmas give you hope, the warmth of Christmas grant you love.

Transition

Any life transition gives us the chance to get in touch with our inner selves.

Transition translates to "change," and most of us are uncomfortable with change; with giving up the familiar and the trusted. But what an opportunity it is to let the fresh and the new in, discovering uncharted territory.

Accepting and embracing change means going with the flow of life; resisting and being fearful means blocking that same flow, and with it, possibly missing out on some incredible new experiences. Someone once said that change is the only constant in life, so we better get used to it and accept it.

As long as we realize that our true inner Self always remains the same, the ebb and flow of life will not affect us negatively and we will have the option to embrace the new roles, knowing that they give us fresh perspective on life and a greater understanding of the lives of others. Remember the saying, "It's the journey, not the destination that matters?"

Personally, I can only say that each time change happened in my life it was scary at first, but looking back I always moved to a better, more exciting place on all levels, physically, emotionally, mentally, spiritually. Embrace transition with joyful anticipation; allow change to happen, but stay true to yourself because that is what life is all about!

The Power of Blessings

A blessing is a prayer, an accepting, an allowing. A blessing raises our vibration by either giving or receiving it. Blessing a person, a situation, or a place means we are putting our attention to it, without judging, wanting or expecting anything; we are creating space.

When we bless someone, we empower that person to prosper, we accept that person in their wholeness. A blessing means making peace with the person or the situation, and it is a simple way of bringing well-being to all those involved.

Lastly and very importantly, a blessing can be a tremendous relief in a situation where letting go is the best option. We have the choice to bless and release a thought, unwanted habit, fear, worry, person, grief, hatred—anything we don't want in our lives.

Remembering

When I look into the eyes of my granddaughter right when she awakens, I see joy and excitement. When my grandson comes running towards me with his arms wide open and a big smile, I see his innocence, his trusting and allowing. There is a familiarity in what I see and a longing. I believe its parts and portions of what I have given away during my life journey; the parts and portions that had to be relinquished in order to be "acceptable," to "fit in."

What if I could recover these treasures? How would my life change if I invited those forgotten gems back? What if my childish innocence and belief in miracles and wonders would return?

Perfection

Being a perfectionist can make life a struggle. But there is a solution to it. Once we realize that we have options, that we have a choice, space opens up for new approaches. It's about acceptance, releasing judgment, and embracing everything in wholeness. Accept the issue/situation as it is, then change it or walk away from it. By starting to accept ourselves from the inside, everything in our outer world will fall into place.

The spiritual journey is not about becoming perfect but to live every moment with awareness, mindfulness and integrity. SSP

IF you believe that you have come to this world to know yourself in all ways and

IF your experience of extremes allows you to know your balance and

IF you choose each commitment of life carefully, with intent and being fully present and doing the best that you are capable of in the moment, then

How can you be anything less than perfect in any category? Gregg Braden, *Walking between the Worlds*

Sacred Union

During the physical union of two people we experience a glimpse of what it feels like when the ego has no agenda. It can be the emptiness of mind that one only experiences in deep meditation.

When there is a deep connection of love, trust and acceptance, physical union can become a sacred moment where control and ego do not matter anymore. There is a merging of higher energies free from our personal feeling of separateness, and we experience a sense of completion. Through sacred relationship/sacred union we can heal our wounds inflicted by the illusion of duality. There is nothing in the universe that love cannot heal.

We need to be courageous, inviting our sacred partner into our life and creating a sacred relationship, even if it takes a long time to happen. Rather than filling our lives with substitutes—overeating, drugs, alcohol, overworking, and so forth—we need to learn to look for the essence of what we are really seeking. Those who are blessed to be in such a relationship or ever had that experience in the past will wholeheartedly agree.

Sacred Moments

There are moments in my life where I am so deeply connected to another being that it is hard to even describe it in worldly terms. Often it happens during a Reiki treatment, when on a level of higher consciousness our spirits meet and connect on a plane that is pure light, acceptance, appreciation and love and dissolve into the vastness of the Universe. Our spirits and souls are engulfed in peace and mutual understanding; no boundaries built by our egos, no judgment or criticism. This is a feeling similar to being deeply and unconditionally in love with someone, or like the moment my children were born where there was nothing but awe and the importance of the present moment. It could even be the honor of being in the holy presence of someone passing away. Those are sacred moments that I deeply cherish and will forever hold in my heart. I feel blessed to have been gifted to experience those precious sacred moments.

A very special and heartfelt THANK YOU, to my children—without you I would have never experienced the sacred moment of giving birth; to my family and friends who "put up with me and all my craziness," to those of you who gave me the opportunity to either teach or do a Reiki treatment with them, giving me the experience of deep trust, connection and healing; to the wonderful friends in my life who allow me to love and cherish them; and to ALL of you who joined me on my sacred journey to live a life worth living—in peace, harmony, love, joy and abundance.

Here is a story of a dear friend of mine about her most sacred moment:

My Most Divine, Sacred Moment

My most Divine, Sacred moment was when my mother was dying from lung cancer and was bedridden at home. It was 12-23-1984. She had turned gray and was in extreme agony. I thought she had passed away and I bent close to her nose to see if I could feel her breath. She startled awake and said "I was there." She said that she had seen the most beautiful white, floaty beings. She said she had never experienced such unconditional love before and was now not afraid of dying anymore. She saw a being and she told "him" that "she wasn't ready to go yet. "I can't die so close to Christmas because of my family." She had "come back" to us when I was close to her nose. She passed away on the 27th AFTER Christmas. She was selfless and didn't want her family to suffer during each holiday season. She was my best friend and soul mate. Because of this, I am not afraid of dying, when it is my time . . . . I would welcome it. She made me realize that death is just another realm of our existence. She gave me unconditional love and hope and courage.

Attitude

"The longer I live, the more I realize the impact of attitude on life. Attitude, to me, is more important than facts. It is more important than the past, the education, the money, than circumstances, than failure, than successes, than what other people think or say or do. It is more important than appearance, giftedness or skill. It will make or break a company . . . a church . . . a home. The remarkable thing is we have a choice everyday regarding the attitude we will embrace for that day. We cannot change our past . . . we cannot change the fact that people will act in a certain way. We cannot change the inevitable. The only thing we can do is play on the one string we have, and that is our attitude. I am convinced that life is 10% what happens to me and 90% of how I react to it. And so it is with you . . . we are in charge of our Attitudes." Charles R Swindoll

Wilderness

The word "Wilderness" is like magic to me. It makes me dream of undisturbed forests, wild rivers, majestic mountains, wild animals. The ring of the word "Wilderness" always has made me tingle all over, and in the wilderness I always find peace and the way to my own heart and soul.

I have traveled the world and there are many lovely places I have seen, visited, experienced; historic places such as the Forum Romano in Rome/Italy, magnificent churches in Italy, France, Germany, beautiful cities, ancient ruins of castles in England, remnants of pre-Colombian artifacts in Colombia. I've seen breathtaking fjords in Norway, swam in tropical waters and traveled the Volga river in Russia. I have stayed in five-star hotels, cozy B&B's. But my most cherished moments are spending the night in the wilderness, curled up in my small backpacking tent or even just sleeping under the stars. I call it my "wilderness therapy." There is a sacred silence to be experienced that does not exist anywhere else, that makes me drink in the oneness with all, the interconnectedness of all beings, trees, mountains, air, water, space. Here it is where I find my happiness, where nothing else matters, where all worries simply vanish. Back to the basics; clean water and air, surrounded only by essentials for survival and yet, profound happiness, contentment and peace are present every second. Living in the moment, watching a bird happily chirping away high in the gently swaying trees above me, listening to the rustling deep in the forest and wondering what animal might be watching me, the soft murmur from the cool, clear stream next to me. Primordial sounds? The origins of mantras? A calmness envelops me like a warm, cozy, familiar blanket. There is nothing else I need right this moment. This is yoga in its essence.

I feel at ease in the backcountry; I know the animals, the elements are my friends. I have slept in a tiny tent above the Arctic Circle where the grizzlies and wolves roam. I have never been afraid in the wilderness. It is said that animals sense fear and that is when they may attack. I believe that they also sense my being comfortable around them, no harmful actions or even thoughts in my mind that could disturb them. In that little tent up in Alaska I felt as safe as in my home in the Colorado mountains. The next morning I discovered huge fresh grizzly tracks not far behind the tent, so the giant had been there during the night, checking me out. I was sound asleep. Being at ease in every situation—that is yoga as well.

Nature

My love of nature began when I was a little, living in Grandma's house with its huge garden full of flowers, fruit trees and veggies. I grew up eating carrots that I just had pulled out of the soil; I picked ripe, juicy berries fresh from the bushes. In the fall the entire family gathered in the garden for the harvest, digging for potatoes, then making a fire and roasting the potatoes right there in the field. These are treasured memories of living in the moment, of healthy food grown not with pesticides, but with lots of love instead.

Nature will always heal and comfort us, no matter what. It is our responsibility to protect and nourish the earth and honor her for all she gives to us. Giving back by stopping pollution in whatever shape or form; it is possible to live in perfect harmony and synergy if we go back to our roots and re-discover what is really important in life.

Last year a dream came true for me by building a greenhouse. After 16 years of unsuccessful gardening at 9,000 feet elevation I finally realized that this is just a continuation of my life path—growing my own food. It was the best decision I have made the last few years. Not only could I feed myself (along with family and friends) for almost six months out of the year with fresh, delicious, organic greens, tomatoes, zucchini, cucumbers, herbs, peppers and carrots, but it was a pleasure working in it as well. No matter what the weather, I was always protected; sometimes storms were raging outside or snow falling, I was safe in my little "plant kingdom." Needless to say that I added another greenhouse this year, which made gardening possible even earlier in March, and I was able to start harvesting in April.

Once again—this is yoga; living in harmony with the environment.

This "working meditation" refreshes me more than anything else. What is it with nature that just simply by being there has such a tremendous impact on us? There is a different vibration, a calming freshness that is rejuvenating and energizing. It is also the stillness that nature provides that is sacred to me. It is sometimes total silence, which actually has its own sound. Yes, the "sound of silence" as one famous song goes. Primordial sounds such as the rushing or gurgling of a stream or river, wind howling on high mountain ridges, the gentle song of falling rain or the tapping of sleet and hail are the healing music nature provides to us for free. Then there are all the stimulating scents of nature; one of my favorites is walking along a sunny trail and suddenly being surrounded by a waft of warm air scented with pine needle aroma; or how about the calming, nurturing smell of rain? In the wintertime, I swear, I can smell when snow is moving in. Mindful-inspired living in full action. Yoga!

I am living my yoga every moment of every day, no matter what I do. When I totally focus on writing—that is yoga. When I wake up in the morning with gratitude in my heart, smiling to myself when I see the rosy morning glow reflecting from the mountains first thing when I open my eyes, when I hear the little bird greeting me with its cheery song, that is yoga. When I fully concentrate on my breathing, drinking in the fresh mountain air deep into my belly, when I completely exhale and let go of any worries that might sneak up, that is yoga.

The Power of Journaling

I had a habit over many years to write into my journal every morning. First thing in the morning I would write down ten things that I am grateful for. It changed my life. Although for the most part it was nothing dramatic, in the common sense and my gratitude has not changed over time. It is the simple things that we mostly take for granted that I express deep daily gratitude for every day:

I am grateful that I had a good night's sleep in a cozy warm bed (just think about how many people on this earth do not have this luxury).

I am grateful that I have a wonderful home (small but beautiful) that is exactly what I need and always wanted, with gorgeous mountain views at 9,000 feet elevation where the air is clean and fresh.

I am grateful to have a good healthy breakfast and am able to grow some of my own food.

I am grateful that I have a wonderful family that lives nearby and we support each other.

I am grateful to have a great circle of friends that have become my soul family.

I am grateful for my good health, vitality and energy.

All of this and so much more to be grateful for and, as you can see, it is not about tons of money, luxurious trips, fancy restaurants and such; it is the simple things in life that matter most and give us the greatest pleasure and contentment.

I have made it a habit to meditate first thing in the morning. This is the only way to start my day and it gives me the calmness, peace and right attitude to go about my day. I just sit up straight in bed, simply close my eyes, take a few deep breaths and allow my mind to relax and release any thoughts, focusing on the breath. As Thich Nhath Hanh says, "When you breathe in breathe in, when you breathe out, breathe out." Sometimes I meditate for an hour, sometimes only five minutes, but I never ever start my day without meditation. Like so many other things in life, it is a matter of habit.

It is said that it takes 21 days to change a habit or to establish a new one. I invite the reader to try this for themselves and expect wonderful things to happen in your life once you establish your own meditation routine.

Simplicity

"Chop wood, carry water," the Buddha once said. What he meant by that is to find enlightenment in simplicity, by developing a deep sense of awareness, a readiness to experience fully whatever comes our way. Living a life in the state of mindfulness, cherishing every moment and being open to discover the good in everything we encounter will help us to find the strength to move from fear to love.

Gratitude

Sitting here at my desk, snow falling in May (this is Colorado after all), a beautiful red fox just hurried through my backyard on its way to catch his dinner. Earlier, a herd of deer was resting below my office window searching shelter from the snow under the sweeping branches of my old, sturdy Ponderosa pine trees. On my morning walk I observed our "resident" herd of bighorn sheep, digesting their sparse breakfast of the few blades of grass that were brave enough to break through the cold soil. I am blessed beyond what I would have ever imagined. I am living in paradise.

Prema (Love)

"Prema" is what my grandkids call me. My grandson "invented" it when he started to speak. The first time I heard him call me Prema it made me cry. Prema means "love" in Sanskrit. What a joy and honor to be given such wonderful name by my little sweetheart.

Love—we all want it, or give it. Most people feel they are not getting enough of it; some think there is nobody who wants their love. For some its romance, others deep commitment, some confuse real love with love-making.

Real love is unconditional, it is just there, as natural as the air we breathe, it is given freely and does not ask anything in return. But what if we give it to someone who does not want our love? It is a painful experience, which most of us have gone through. We don't understand why someone would reject being loved. Is it that they are afraid of losing control if they allow to be loved, as someone once explained to me?

Loving someone who does not want our love is a hard thing to swallow. I am speaking from experience. It is one of my most significant growing experiences I have gone through and it has changed the way I think, respond, and react. I realized that no matter how much we love someone it is not about us. I have given to this relationship all I have, I sacrificed, I pleaded, I forgave, I disregarded what I needed. I was willing to change and bend backwards because I loved this person so much, but my mistake was to expect love, respect, and commitment in return. It was NOT unconditional love as I thought it was. It was a combination of love, romance, attraction, passion, and lust! It was a very rocky few years that made me realize that I was not doing this person justice, nor myself. I realize that all the issues, flaws and betrayals were learning experiences I could have walked away from a long time ago. I chose not to. I chose to suffer through it with the hope that time and I could change things. That is pure ego involvement; I know this now. What I also learned and realized is that I need to love and respect myself, because if I don't then how can I expect someone else to love and respect me? We always have choices; we can accept a situation, change it or walk away from it. It is always up to us. I am now grateful for having had this experience; it was a steep and painful learning curve but it was worth it and it made me grow and move forward on my dharmic path.

I live alone, but I am not lonely. I have the most amazing and fulfilling relationships in my life with a supportive, extraordinary family and a large circle of wonderful friends. I am surrounded by love and light wherever I go and I love my life the way it is. Yes, it would be terrific to share it with a likeminded soul but if not, so be it. I am still happy. Life is good, life is great. An unknown, yet very insightful, person once wrote, "I haven't lived an ordinary life and I am not starting now!" Life is as good as we make it. I have choices. I can appreciate all the wonders and miracles that are all around me all the time if I open my eyes, ears, and most importantly my heart. Or I can choose not to—but it's up to me. I choose to expect miracles every day, and surely they arrive. "When one door closes another one will surely open," my dad used to say to me when I was little. And how right he was; but sometimes we stare at the door that just shut in front of us so long and with such intensity that we miss the one that opens elsewhere. Going with the flow, keeping a light heart and not taking things too seriously makes life so much easier.

I am in love—with my life! I love my family, friends, my home, the beautiful state and country I live in and that I have dreamed about for a long time. I made it happen. I am here now. I love my garden, the mountains, and the wild animals that visit with me on a daily basis. I love my career, my students. I love my body, mind and spirit. Little things can inspire me and make me smile; like my friend the fox, who accompanies me on my morning walks. The sun breaking through the clouds on a rainy day like today reminds me that light and love are always there even when they are sometimes hidden form our view.

I feel very fortunate for the life that was given to me, with all its challenges, ups and downs; all of it made me who I am now. There were times when I hit bottom. I thought it was the end of everything but when I realized that everything moves according to a Divine plan, which works in ebbs and flows, with rising high and falling low, with growth and decay, hardships and happiness I found peace. Allowing this natural flow to just happen, to actually embrace whatever comes along I found harmony.

About Loss—Navajo—A Dog's Life

Our once "family dog" crossed over the rainbow bridge today. We got him when we first came to Bailey, Colorado 16 years ago as an eight-week-old puppy. He came with us to England and survived their cruel quarantine regimen before we all moved back to Bailey. He lived a happy life with four other dogs and my son and daughter-in-law. He died peacefully in the place he loved and was surrounded by "his" people. A sad day nevertheless. Love and peace to you, Navajo.

It was a bitter cold snowy November evening when I saw a post on a local website that someone had a litter of Siberian Huskies and was looking for homes for some of them. I had made a promise to my son that he would get a dog in our new home here in Colorado. I showed him the ad and asked if he wanted to take a look at the puppies. His beaming smile was the answer. We called and the owners said they had two puppies left. We were dressed and in the car in minutes. It was a long drive from Bailey all the way down to Turkey creek. The roads were icy, it was a pitch-dark night, and a blizzard making driving hazardous—nevertheless, we were determined. When we knocked on the door a ferocious bark from the other side greeted us and scared me half to death, which was the mom we learned later. The owner let us in and we got the first look of "our" little dog. What a precious cute ball of fur with the biggest paws, the bluest eyes, the softest fur. Love at first site for all of us.

We stopped for dog food on the way home, my son cradling and keeping his puppy warm in his jacket. Another long, slow drive home, where we found a box and blankets for the little guy and settled for the night. Nobody got much sleep, though. "Navajo" as we named him later, was missing his mom, dad and brother and cried all night long.

The next day we found out that by coincidence our neighbor had adopted Navajo's little brother. What a joy to watch the two of them play together again! It made the transition so much easier, but it also meant that any chance he got, he would "escape" out of the fenced yard to go play with his sibling.

It's easy to love a little puppy, even for me who has always been very afraid of dogs. I did not grow up with animals and they felt like a threat to me. Navajo cured me of that fear with his trust and his playfulness. When the kids had to go to school Navajo and I went on long hikes together. He made me feel safe and he looked "scary" to some people just because of his size he eventually grew into. Being a mix of Siberian Husky and Norwegian Elkhound, running and pulling was in his blood, so hiking was not always easy. Uphill was fun as he actually pulled us up; downhill—another story. After he was grown we took him ski joring and dog sledding, which he enjoyed tremendously and so did we. But not all was glory in his little life.

The time came when we had to move to England, which had a very strict quarantine law at that time. But we had no choice. The kennel was a two-hour drive from where we lived and he had to stay there for six months. I drove to see him almost five days a week and we sat on the rough concrete floor together. At first when I came he was jumping up and down smiling his big doggie smile, I could actually hear him bark his welcome from way down the road, he knew I was coming. We played with his toys and he got his little bit of exercise in that cruel small space of maybe 3x10feet of fenced dog run. But soon his eyes would turn sad and he would lay down right in front of the door as to say, "please, don't leave me." It was heartbreaking to see him, the "runner of the wild" like that. I cried each time I had to leave and I heard him whine long after I had left the kennel. Of course, during the weekends the entire family went to see him and the same scenario happened—from happiness to despair, for all of us.

Finally the six months quarantine time was over and the day arrived when we could pick Navajo up and bring him home. Luckily our home was a typical "Cotswold" British stone home with a walled garden and he could play, run, jump and romp as much as he liked. His wild spirit and the smile in his face returned quickly. We took him on long walks, always on a leash though as he had never really been able to be trained. We tried the training—especially me, the one who had no previous experience with dogs… so I had him on a leash and had my daughter give him the "come, stay" etc. commands. Well, it turned out he was a fast learner. She said "come" once and he pulled so hard on the leash that he caught me by surprise and dragged me belly down through the goose poop along the shores of the nearby lake. Lots of laughter from my daughter and a surprised look from our pup! The next training sessions took place in the walled garden and we thought we had it all figured out. Navajo seemed to learn the commands and to obey. Next step, we took him on a walk along the Thames River through the wide-open fields. Carefully we took off the leash and tried the commands. It worked for a while until he realized that there was more to discover and that the leash was "really" gone. He took off like a daredevil and an entire family chasing after him. Soon we lost sight of him, so we scattered in all directions to find him. I heard a whimper in the distance; there were hedges and large tangled blackberry bushes. Could it be that he got stuck there? Sure enough that's where he was; whining, shaking, lost. He was so happy to see me but unable to get out. Down on my belly I went again, crawling through the thorny blackberry bushes, eventually getting a hold of him and crawling back out—on all fours. Gotta' love your dog…

On a trip to Wales the little rascal almost tore my arm out while I had him on the leash, hiking in the hills when a rabbit jumped out in front of us, and what would any decent dog do? Of course, he tried to chase the rabbit. I held on to the leash after all our off-leash experiences and ended up with a severe rotator cuff injury—but I still loved him.

Luck had it that our stay in England was not supposed to last very long and happily we returned back to Bailey, regretting what we had to put Navajo through with quarantine. But home, at last. Freedom!

My son spent several months building a log doghouse for Navajo, cutting the trees from our property, hand-peeling them and putting it all together. The doghouse was fancier than our cabin that we lived in. We spent evenings around the campfire with Navajo in our laps under the deep dark blue Colorado night sky. We went on long hikes again together enjoying nature, open space and beauty all around us. On one particular hike we decided to take our lunch break in a beautiful Aspen grove. Normally Navajo would lay down as soon as we would sit for our break. Not so this time. He nervously ran from side-to-side, not wanting to settle down. We knew something was not right and decided to trust his instincts. We got up and continued hiking a little further, where we were surrounded by bluebirds. Of course I needed to capture them on film; clicking away with my camera I happened to look back to the place where we wanted to eat our lunch to see a black bear coming right out of it. Thank you Nav (our abbreviation for "Navajo"): you may have saved our lives.

We spent many wonderful years with him camping, hiking, fishing, playing. When my son got married and had his own home and family Navajo went with him, but it was not far from me and we all could be together on a regular basis.

Navajo's wild youthful energy slowly faded over the years and he turned into a mellow, sometimes a bit grumpy old dog—just like us humans change over the course of our lives.

Navajo came into our lives on a bitter cold winter night. Today, on a beautiful warm summer day, the day of the Summer Solstice, Navajo decided that it was time to move on to another dimension. He had lived 16 happy years, without any major illnesses (except a broken leg a few years ago), and with four other companion dogs in a huge yard. It was his time to say good-bye. Accepting death is not easy, but dying in a wonderful place like he did is a privilege. We made him as comfortable as possible, he lay on the deck in a light breeze, shaded by a large umbrella, surrounded by his human family and his little animal family of Gretchen, Bruno, Heidi and the two cats; even the rooster was singing him a good-bye song.

I had lost my Tibetan Terrier puppy a few years ago. Saddhu was only ten-weeks-old when he died in my arms; he had parvo (a deadly disease that kills young puppies). I will never forget how he was clinging to me when we sat at the animal hospital and I had no other option as to have him put down to end his suffering. I remember his big eyes that had turned all grey and dull, his soft glossy fur that had lost its entire luster and how his body went limp when he crossed over. All those memories came back today and along with them the pain that I felt back then.

Many gentle hands where stroking Navajo today. I invoked some Reiki energy to help with the transition, and in the late afternoon Navajo let out his last breath and peacefully crossed the rainbow bridge.

It was hard to watch him slowly fading, but it was even harder seeing my son grieve over the loss of his longtime companion and friend, the first dog he had ever had and the special connection with him. It breaks a mother's heart to see their children suffer and it broke mine, but I feel honored that I was present during those moments and maybe a comfort for both of them.

FINAL NOTES

Writing has become a meditation and inspiration in itself. Meditation—because I become completely absorbed and focused through the process. I forget to eat, what time it is or to take a break. Inspiration—because reliving my life this way is like an epiphany to discover what is possible, how to overcome obstacles, how to really live life to the fullest without regrets, and to hopefully give the courage to the reader to believe in themselves when times get tough. In turn, this courage will hopefully inspire you, the reader, to keep going, to start over, to never give up, to keep your gaze inward, and to see the silver lining within yourself, not at a distant horizon. It's all here inside of you, it's in the here and now.

I am by no means an expert. I have not studied with any famous yoga teachers, and I have never been to India or any places in Asia for that matter, which these days seem to be the pre-requisite to become a respected yogini. Instead, I followed my own path guided by my heart and inspiring books of accomplished teachers, and taking classes to advance my yoga practice and to further develop my spirituality. There has always been the beacon of truthfulness, faith and "can-do" attitude for me. I studied with different teachers (some of them probably as good as today's famous yoga icons) but it has never been important to me how famous someone is. What matters to me is the fact that a person is walking their talk, has a compassionate loving heart, and the true desire to help others. I have found those qualities in my teachers, whether real living human beings or enlightened masters that have long passed but nevertheless have guided me with their wisdom through deep insights and scriptures.

We all have to find our own personal path. We need the power, faith and trust into our own judgment to determine which way is right for us, and luckily that is different for everyone. Allowing our hearts to guide us with love and understanding and appreciating the flow of life with all its ups and downs transforms life into the richest experience we could ever ask for. An inspired life is a life that embraces everything encountered, whether good or bad. Over time we will find the balance, and what once appeared good may not seem that way anymore; and to the contrary, what had looked bad might turn out to be the best thing that's ever happened. "Stay in the center of the circle and let all things take their course," the Dalai Lama said—***that*** is the true way of an inspired life.

I encourage you, the reader, to take a deep and long look at your life. Look at it as the observer, like looking from the outside.

What do you see? Do you see a life rich in experiences, full of love, abundance, happiness? If not, look deeper. It is all there. It may be concealed at first, like clouds hiding the sun and beautiful blue sky; but it's all there for you to uncover. Just open your eyes, your heart and your soul and take what is your birthright—unbounded happiness. Let's walk on this inspiring dharmic path to bliss together.

Namaste (The Divine in me honors the Divine in You)
Sophia

YOGA STUDENT'S STORIES

Lexi Miller

Yoga has changed my life in many ways. When I first started practicing yoga I had terrible anxiety; it was hard to focus during meditation, and the poses never seemed to feel comfortable or "right." I thought that maybe I wasn't cut out for yoga although I still enjoyed the feeling and relaxation I received from the practice. I continued onward, hoping to gain more flexibility. After a couple weeks I felt the stretches and their benefits, and breathing, meditation and yoga all seemed to fit together and make sense to me. I began applying meditation to my daily life and during stressful situations. When I meditate, I imagine all things good entering my lungs and filling up my body, and all negative things leaving. I realized that meditating when I had anxiety helped me gain control of it. Saying mantras is another way I gained relief. Anxiety is something I have had to live with for many years, and yoga has helped me open up and let go of many of the worries I had.

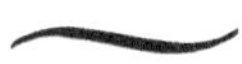

Sondra Spratta

...My sister has been telling me for years that yoga is the best thing one can do for the body and mind. I have suffered from headaches my entire life and it is very hard for me to sit still and relax long enough to enjoy yoga. I have tried to do yoga tapes at home in by living room, but I never practiced long enough to get hooked. I thought if I enrolled in this class

I would be "forced" to commit to yoga, and could then I could decide if it was something I wanted to continue.

My experience so far has been enjoyable, and I think regular yoga could lessen the chance for injury during activity. First and foremost, I looked for this class to stretch and reflect. Yoga is not for the weak, whether it's weakness in the body or the mind. Low-impact strengthening is the best kind, and strong muscles to support structure are important to my individual health and wellness in the future. ... For me personally, it is much more about the very basic muscle health and support. However, I always love to learn whatever the direction of growth.

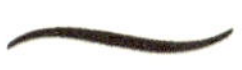

Thuy Nguyen

I had never imagined myself attending a yoga class or wanting to learn yoga. Working two jobs and focusing on a 3.0 GPA can weaken a person's astral body, and I commonly felt unmotivated to do much else. After attending a couple sessions, I used some of the methods taught to relax. One of my favorites is Savasana, because I can lay there unmoving and fully relaxed, and go into a deep relaxation. Bringing yoga into my chaotic lifestyle helps me improve many things in my lifestyle, from my sleeping habits to diet to anger issues. Before going to sleep, I try to do four sun salutations and a few warrior pose; this helps me stay in a deep sleep and then I am fully restored the next morning.

Half of my family members are Buddhists and we attend the Vietnamese Buddhist temple weekly where meditation is practiced often at the shrine. But for me, it's easier to relax with spiritual musical beats than a group of monks chanting aloud. The spiritual music tends to clear my mind, and my breathing flows smoothly. I started eating healthier, and one of the monks told me that soybean is very good for your skin and can reduce acne. Eating more vegetables and drinking tons of water has helped my body build a strong immune system, making it less vulnerable to sickness or disease.

Learning yoga gave me an advantage to life; learning how to take control gave me a method of balancing myself with the world.

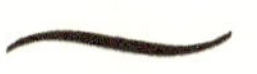

Josh Hildebrand, RRCC yoga student

As a practicing yoga student for a short time now, I find that while meditating, mantras and mudras, if used properly, allow me to gain control over my body and mind. My mind tends to wander during meditation, but by chanting and using my hands it allows me to focus. These are definitely a huge aspect of my meditation practices and it's my belief that every student of yoga should study further to understand the power that these mantras and mudras can carry with them.

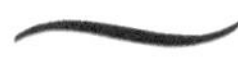

Jake Spencer

. . . . yoga entails a lot more than I expected.

First off, I had no idea that yoga had so much to do with breathing.

When I first heard this, I was a bit skeptical so I did not breathe the the way it was taught in yoga. After a few classes I decided to try letting my breath initiate the movement, and breathe along with it. There was an immediate difference in the way the poses felt, and it quickly became easier and felt more natural for me. Furthermore, I find that concentrating on your breath is something that actually takes effort. Most of us go along our day-to-day lives not even thinking about breathing because our bodies do it naturally. But when you take the time out to focus on breathing it has a way of relaxing you.

The other thing that surprised me about yoga is that there is a whole lifestyle that goes along with it. It was cool to discover the **Yamas** and **Niyamas**, and how people who embrace the yogic lifestyle incorporate them into their lives, including diet. And the concept of karma is not something I knew to be related to yoga. Though I do not believe in karma myself, it was good to learn about what others believe and that it is associated with the yogic lifestyle.

As far as the poses and movement go, some are easier than expected and others have been much harder than I ever thought. For example, I never would have thought there would be a pose as simple as putting your legs up a wall, I never imagined how hard multiple sun salutations could be, and even though I regularly exercise my abs, the boat poses were quite difficult.

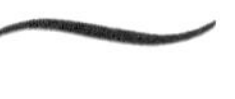

Denise White

Walking into yoga class this semester, I was confident because I already knew some of the poses. But I was also nervous because the yoga I took in high school involved a lot of flexibility, which I have little of. Even though it was a wonderful introduction to yoga, I can look back and see that it was a more advanced level of stretching than I possess even now. However, Sophia's class has been very easy and gentle compared with that one. I feel like I am able to move at my own pace and not have to worry about fitting in with everyone else's flexibility levels. In this class I feel like I can really understand and work my way slowly into the poses that we learn, gradually making my way up to the harder ones and developing a better relationship with this form of exercise.

I have had much experience with meditation and aligning my chakras from my own spiritual practices, but doing savasana along with the poses has made it that much more relaxing, and somehow empowering. I can feel my body getting stronger every time I do yoga, and feel like the practices are slowly becoming unconsciously incorporated into my day-to-day life. After yoga, my muscles feel awake, charged with energy, and my whole body relaxed in a way that nothing else can mimic. My favorite pose, the sun salutation, embodies this. It is truly an amazing sensation, and one that I am very thankful to know and enjoy learning. I am so glad that I have gotten back into classes, because they have renewed that rush of inner peace inside me that opens up every time I do yoga.

Elise Austin

Yoga is known for being relaxing, calming, and bringing balance into one's life. What I *didn't* realize is that yoga is also difficult and challenging. It is above all though rewarding. Yoga came as quite a surprise to me when I started taking the class, and then the more I practiced outside of class, the more rewarding it became. There is a sense of accomplishment after completing a repeated set of poses that are challenging. Energy levels are increased, mood is lifted—there is just a general sense of peace in the body and mind. I tried to practice the breathing exercises everywhere I went, especially when I had anxiety. I wanted to really understand the concept of yoga, balancing my body, mind and spirit, since my mind always seemed to be racing. By taking a short break during a quiz to close my eyes and concentrate on my breathing, it made a world of difference for my concentration, awareness, and my anxiety levels. So far, yoga has dramatically changed my life and it is just the beginning. What I love best about this whole journey is learning that I don't necessarily need medication to solve my problems. I can do it myself, with concentration and determination. I have always strived for balance in every part of my life, and I think yoga significantly helps me get closer to my ultimate goal of harmony.

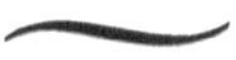

Dustin Lund

The last fifteen years of my life have been a roller coaster ride, one that I didn't think I would ever get off of. It was go-go-go from sunrise to sunset, with no time for myself. I wasn't necessarily using all the hours of the days productively; I was just filling my days with things to do.

I was involved in a serious accident and it took me a year and a half to realize that life might be worth living. I found a couple of jobs that got me by, but with no real sense of purpose or direction.

The first day of yoga class seemed totally strange to me. Looking in the mirror at the studio, I realized I was about a foot taller than everybody else and wasn't sure yoga was going to be for me. But the first five weeks of yoga class grew on me.

Now I do some yoga two or three days a week and it is "me time." I am learning how important breathing is, particularly with meditation, and learning how I can become less scattered mentally to develop some focus and have purpose in my daily actions.

I am finding that I feel better as a person and am taking time to think about my actions instead of just running on instinct and making spur of the moment decisions. Making spur of the moment decisions has led me to some stupid results in the past, and I would like to get out of that habit.

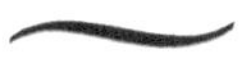

Kelsey Wood

I decided to try yoga because my husband and I became intrigued with the Buddhist way of life. Before taking this class I associated yoga mainly with Buddhism, and then I learned that yoga encompasses and includes *all* religion. That is now one of my favorite parts of the yoga experience, because I've always believed in co-existence. I feel like I've only scratched the surface of the yogic lifestyle, but I am definitely going to continue my exploration.

I used to be pretty laid back and slow to anger, but having a child seemed to change that drastically. I enrolled in this class hoping that it would help relieve stress and be more patient with my 2 ½ year old son. Along with regular exercise, the techniques I've learned for meditation, and focusing on my breathing to clear my mind, my hopes are being fulfilled! I even believe my concentration and focus has improved. Instead of feeling anxious and irritated so easily, I've been able to breathe and assess the situation more clearly before reacting. For me, yoga has been a great stress relief.

Meditation is a new concept for me. At first I wasn't sure what I was doing, or if I was doing it right. Then I saw the benefits: clearing my mind entirely and just being able to feel into my body. This is probably where my increased focus and concentration came from. Each time I meditate I seem to be able to keep my mind calmer and clearer then the time before—not an easy feat for me.

Kendra Alexandria Bartholomew

What brought me to yoga? I was initially very nervous about my non-existent skill level, but quickly learned that is not what it is about. It was about making my best effort, and being reassured that the strength and stamina would come. I did not find the poses difficult, for the most part, but I did realize areas that definitely could use some strengthening. With the ease that I felt with the movements, I had no idea how much I was working my body. It was amazing, to feel my body gathering strength. It was never that sore, aching, painful experience I've had from an intense work out. It was a breath of fresh air for me. I felt my energy coming back, and continued on my own with the practice.

One of the things I appreciate most about yoga is the acceptance is there at all skill levels. In other physical activities, there is usually a sense of competition and constant comparison. With yoga, it's come as you are and perform to the best of your ability. The idea is that if you fail today, it will only make you stronger tomorrow. An empowering statement! There is so much support and reassurance that everyone has gone through it, everyone will make it through, and everyone will be stronger through their practice.

Faith Craver, My Yogic Practice

… after taking Yoga One, I realized that the practice comes in many different forms.

. . . In yoga, the breathing alone is a magnificent stress relief and can be a completely personal experience. I find that after every yoga class, I feel lighter, relieved and also happier. Being the positive person that I am, yoga attracted me and now I can't picture my life without it.

After that first yoga class, I was captivated. I loved how peaceful the setting felt and immediately wanted to progress in the practice. I feel like yoga will not only be a tool I can use to help me through college, but also one that can help me throughout life. Yoga can help me grow in patience and be a better person. I have a new hobby that I enjoy, a way to relieve stress, a form of exercise that does not torture my body, and a new profound and deeper connection with my own being . . . . I know that I will continue to practice yoga, and that I will draw others into the practice as well.

Emilee Roman, Reflection on Yoga

To me, the most important part of yoga is the feeling you have once you've completed a session. At the beginning, my body feels tight and weak. As I move through the poses and breathe deeply from my nose to my toes, (this is what I say to myself throughout my practice to affirm that my asthma and problems with circulation won't hinder me) I feel the strength building in my body. This confidence in your own ability is something that will carry you through life, and yoga is where I get this confidence the most. The feeling of peace and inner strength after a yoga class is what makes me want to go back for more.

… I feel calmer and more in control when I practice yoga.

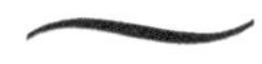

Blake Collins, Meditation

Sitting calmly I deeply stir my breath and inhale. Conscious and award of my surroundings I push the air out. With each breath I become more and more relaxed, focused, and aware. My consciousness in focused, like a stream of water through a funnel. This energy is powerful, warm, pure. It illuminates my mind and unites my mind, body and soul. In this meditative state I am, and am not.

... Our minds have practically become strangers to the bodies they inhabit. Meditation is a way back in. It is a way to rediscover ourselves as moral and rational beings. By sitting and doing very little, our minds are capable of great things. By practicing meditation we can return to what it means to be a part of nature.

Meditation is an inward journey that must be made with pure intentions. We live in the most stimulating era the world has ever seen. Meditation is more important now than it has ever been. It is all too easy to get lost in the material aspect of today's society. Positive endeavors such as meditation help to keep us grounded in what it means to be human.

Yoga is your own return to nature; to your alignment with the Divine and the awareness of the present moment. Being in alignment translates into being in the flow, the flow of life, the flow of nature, the flow of our own true essence. Yoga can be calming or energizing; it can make us more focused and in tune with our own life path. Yoga can make us more compassionate towards others and ourselves, and it can open new pathways on our very own, beautiful personal journey. Yoga will make us healthier over time on all levels, mentally, emotionally, physically and spiritually. Yoga will clear the channels for us to connect to our own spirituality and the spirit of the universe. Yoga infuses our bodies, minds and souls with what is our innate joy and happiness that we all tend to forget or lose over the course of our lives. Yoga is a way to re-connect and re-discover all aspects of our true human nature. Yoga simply will make the world a better place for all to be in it.

If we keep our intentions fresh, clear and inspiring, even in the face of internal or external obstacles; when we look for the journey as the destination and enjoy and deeply cherish every moment or path, we know we have chosen the right direction.

Elizabeth Anna Okino DeVere, Co-Founder of OneDropWithinTheWave.com

Consciousness is Supreme Presence, the calm poise of thought, feeling and action in any given moment. Destructive behavior of any sort shall not thrive where consciousness resides.

I began meditating twice a day, half an hour in the morning, half an hour in the evening, ever conscious of the movement of my breath in and out. The inner peace, and moments of harmony began to expand beyond my morning meditation session, and well into the rest of my day. Bringing my conscious attention to the movement of my breath throughout the day brought the harmony of my meditation into every aspect of every day. I was practicing the living meditation.

What was first a stretching work out, that any gymnast or dancer could do, evolved into a dance with God, a celebration of Unity. Now, I practice breathing through different Yoga asanas every day, whether it be for ten minutes, or 90 minutes. The practice of Yoga allows me the experience, of resting in the balance point between outer and the inner, the point from which all creation takes place, that place of total awareness, harmony experienced. I have found myself quite naturally incorporating simple asanas, and conscious breathing exercises at different points throughout the day, helping me re-center, after or while working at the computer, or after listening to someone express anger or sorrow. The conscious attention to the breath, applied throughout the day, whether walking, stretching, working, or sitting, is The Living Yoga, experienced; the eternal dance with the Divine, Great Spirit, the Mighty I Am Presence, God, and it is this form this glorious place of Presence, of Conscious Awareness that Life is meant to be lived. Namaste.

Jacob Daniel Okino DeVere, Co-Founder of OneDropWithinTheWave.com

I had a much different perspective of yoga when I unknowingly started discovering my spiritual path. Allowing my own personal yoga to bubble up from within, collect in my heart and consciously guide my every thought, word and action—these were not what I expected. My first perspective, which was shared widely among Western men, was that Yoga was basically for sissies who couldn't, or chose not to, play competitive contact sports.

It is safe to say that I did not instantly awaken to the gift hidden within yoga. Then meditation entered my life on a wave, showing me a stillness, that calm golden core of Energy that I had tapped into while playing soccer when "in the zone." Yoga evolved from a workout and something physical into something mental, which allowed for becoming calm and centered.

My introduction to Anusara Yoga gave me great insight into this seemingly invisible connection to the Divine. When I considered, "What is Yoga to me?" I came to a deeper understanding. The natural expansion of yoga in one's life, or any spiritual practice for that matter, is to completely fill one's life with the practice. I had never thought about it, yoga, "completely" filling my life. In an attempt to understand what that could mean, my imagination produced an image of what life would be like "filled" with yoga: every breath conscious, every movement deliberate. Then I realized, yoga has been the physical preparation for existing within the awakened or enlightened state of being consciously aware of our connection with and the presence of God, and our union with the Divine. Shortly after this the "Living Yoga" and the "Heart Breath" came forth. Breathe through the Heart as often as possible to experience Peace and true Happiness, and may all paths be showered with blessings and wondrous awakening.

BIBLIOGRAPHY/RECOMMENDED READING/RESOURCES

Ashley Farrand, Thomas. *Healing Mantras.* New York: Random House, 1999; ISBN 0-345-43170-7

Chodron, Pema. *Start Where You Are.* Boston: Shambala,1994; ISBN-13: 978-1590301425

Chopra, Deepak. *The Spontaneous Fulfillment of Desire.* New York: Harmony books, 2003; ISBN 0-609-60042-7

Clason, George S. *The Richest Man in Babylon.* New York: Penguin Group, 1988; ISBN 0-451-20536-7

Desikachar, T.K.V. *The Heart of Yoga.* Rochester: Inner Transitions International, 1999; ISBN 0-89281-764-X

Devi, Nischala Joy. *The Secret Power of Yoga.* New York: Three Rivers Press, 2007; ISBN-978-0-307-33969-0

Francis, John. *The Ragged Edge of Silence.* Washington D.C.: National Geographic, 2011; ISBN 978-1-4262-0723-5

Gilbert, Elizabeth. *Eat, Pray, Love.* New York: Penguin Books, 2006; ISBN 978-0-14-303841-2

Hay, Louise. *Heal your Body.* Carlsbad: Hay House, 1982; ISBN 0-937611-00-X

Halevi, Peggy. *The Art of Appreciation.* Halevi Publishing, 2009; ISBN 978-0984328802

Hanson Lasater, Judith. *Living your Yoga.* Berkley: Rodnell Press, 2000; ISBN 978-0962713880

Harrell, Keith. *Attitude is Everything.* New York: Harper Business, 2005; ISBN-10: 0060779721

Harvey, Andrew. *Heat Yoga.* Berkeley: North Atlantic Books, 2010; ISBN-13: 978-1556438974

Harvey, Andrew. *The Hope.* United States: Hay House, 2009; ISBN 978-1-4019-2003-6

Hill, Napoleon. *Think and Grow Rich.* New York: Facet Crest, 1960; ISBN 0-449-21492-3

Hirschi, Gertrud. *Mudras.* Maine: Red Wheel/Weiser, LLC, 2000; ISBN 1-57863-139-4

Judith, Anodea. *Eastern Body/Western Mind.* Berkeley: Celestial Arts, 1996; ISBN1-58761-225-9

Kempton, Sally. *Meditation for the Love of it.* Boulder: Sounds True, Inc, 2011; ISBN-13: 978-1604070811

Kraftsow, Gary. *Yoga for Transformation.* New York: Penguin Compass, 2002; ISBN-13: 978-0140196290

Levine, Stephen. *Guided Meditations.* New York: Anchor books Double Day, 1991; ISBN 0-385-41737-3

MSI. *Enlightenment.* Waynesville: SFA Publications, 1996; ISBN-13: 978-0931783173

Rama, Swami. *The Art of Joyful Living.* Honesdale: Himalayan Institute Press, 2003; ISBN-13: 978-0893892364

Rama, Swami. *Meditation and its Practice.* Honesdale: Himalayan Institute Press, 1992 ISBN-13: 978-0893891534

Ravi Ravindera. *The Spiritual Roots of Yoga*. Sandpoint: Morning Light Press, 2006; ISBN-13: 978-1596750111

Salzberg, Sharon. *A Heart as Wide as the World.* Boston and London: Shambala, 1999; ISBN-13: 978-1570624285

Salzberg, Sharon. *Loving-Kindness*. Boston and London: Shambala, 2002; ISBN-13: 978-1590305577

Salzberg, Sharon. *Real Happiness*. New York: Workman Publishing, 2011; ISBN-13: 978-0761159254

Schiffman, Erich. *Moving into Stillness*. New York: Pocket Books, 1996; ISBN 0-671-53480-7

Sell, Christina. *Yoga from the Inside Out*. Prescott: Hohm Press, 2003; ISBN-13: 978-1890772321

Shunryu, Suzuki. *Zen Mind, Beginner's Mind.* New York and Tokyo: Weatherhill, 1974; ISBN-13: 978-1590308493

Thich Nhat Hanh. *The Heart of the Buddha's Teaching.* Berkeley: Broadway Books, 1999; ISBN-13: 978-0767903691

Thich Nhat Hanh. *Chanting from the Heart*. Berkeley: Parallax Press, 2006; ISBN-13: 978-1888375633

Thich Nhat Hanh. *The Blooming of a Lotus*. Boston: Beacon Press, 2009; ISBN 978-0-8070-1238-3

Tolle, Eckhard. *The Power of Now*. Novato: New World Library, 2004; ISBN 978-1577314806

Williamson, Marianne. *Enchanted Love*. New York: Touchstone, 1999; ISBN 0-684-84219-X

Williamson, Marianne. *Illuminata*. New York: Random House, 1994; ISBN-13: 978-1573225205

Ziglar, Zig. *Better Than Good.* Nashville: Thomas Nelson, 2006; 9-781-59145-400-7

YOGA TERMINOLOGY

Namaste (also called Anjali Mudra or Prayer position)
Asana practice (the physical yoga poses)
Hatha yoga (The word "hatha" comes from the Sanskrit terms "ha" meaning "sun" and "tha" meaning "moon". Hatha Yoga is known as the branch of Yoga that unites pairs of opposites referring to the positive (sun) and negative (moon) currents in the system. Wikipedia)
Mantras (sacred transformational words used in meditation)
Mudras (hand positions)
Vipashyana meditation (insight meditation)
Prana (life force)
Shushumna (central channel, similar to the spine)
Chakras (energy centers in our bodies)
Savasana (corpse pose, relaxation at end of yoga class)
Naturopathy (a form of alternative medicine based on a belief in vitalism)
Reiki (energy healing modality)
Shoshoni (yoga retreat center)
Pranayama (controlled breathing)
Seva (selfless service)
Samsara (literally means "wandering on")

Om Namah Shivaya (popular mantra in Shaivism)
Sangha (spiritual community)
Dharma (spiritual life path)
Anjali Mudra (hands placed in prayer position in front of the heart)
Ahimsa (non violence)
Yamas/Niyamas (rules of living)

For further information please visit

www.sophiapaul.com

www.royalyogabailey.com

For information on OmShanti Yoga Wear—eco conscious, custom, handmade yoga wear please visit www.omshantiyogawear.com

www.ingramcontent.com/pod-product-compliance
Lightning Source LLC
Chambersburg PA
CBHW020412290526
45785CB00002B/526

9781452539966